WHAT PEOPLE
TARA HEATON

MW01088005

"Raw and unapologetically real, *Life Minutes* is like a power-walk with your best friend. Tara Heaton's words are a dagger and a balm to the heart where the refusal to identify as a victim defines radical resilience. It's an unforgettable memoir of fiery hope, tenacious wit, and unwavering maternal devotion — a risk-taker's battle cry to love."

— Madeleine Goforth
Screenwriter, Actor, Storyteller

"Tara Heaton is a writer with courage, determination, insight, wisdom, and love. The immediacy of her words invited me into a dangerous journey and kept me there. She has risen and transformed the ravages of heartbreak and despair. She shares her story with unabashed forthrightness, and I am moved beyond words."

— Pam Noble
Author, Poet, Mother

To Kim
w/ joy & gratitude

LIFE
MINUTES

Igniting Joy from
the Fire of Heartache

A TRUE STORY

TARA HEATON

Life Minutes

For information about this title or to order other books and/or electronic media, contact the publisher:

Two Sisters Writing & Publishing®
TwoSistersWriting.com
18530 Mack Avenue, Suite 166
Grosse Pointe Farms, MI 48236

Hardcover ISBN: 978-1-956879-74-2
Paperback ISBN: 978-1-956879-75-9
Ebook ISBN: 978-1-956879-76-6

Printed in the United States of America

No part of this manuscript is fiction. Only some names of people and places have been changed. No part of this book was written with AI assistance.

Book cover art and design: Penny Treese.
Graphics and formatting: Illumination Graphics.
Author photos: The Heaton Family Collection.

I promised my children that their suffering would not be wasted, that we would make it matter. This book is me, making good on that promise. It is my greatest desire that when you close this book, you are able to live with more freedom, more light, and a deeper ability to love and be loved. If *Life Minutes* awakens a flame that says you are the dictator of your joy factor, your spirit, then it will have served its purpose.

—Tara Heaton

DEDICATION

To every mom. From my heart to yours.

CONTENTS

A FLAME

August 1975. I was a rising fourth grader, enamored with ballet, *Little House on the Prairie* books, and David Cassidy. I also loved being the only sister to an older and a younger brother. During the summers, we spent most of our days in the water at Murraywood pool in Irmo, South Carolina, only hitting the deck when the whistle blew and the lifeguard yelled, "Adult swim!"

My brothers and I would race over to our mom where she bathed in an aromatic bubble of Hawaiian Tropic, Lark cigarettes, and Diet Pepsi. With bright-colored beach towels, we dried off enough to take a bologna sandwich or a Little Debbie oatmeal cream pie from Mom's carefully-packed cooler.

On this particular day, it was nearing dinner time, but Mom hadn't packed an afternoon snack. We were happy to be hungry, because our dad was coming to the pool after golf, and we were going out to dinner.

The crowd began to clear as the lifeguards stacked chairs and rolled up lane ropes. The last dozen kids were gathered in the deep end, lined up at the high dive where we could splash into the 12 feet of chlorine-clean blue water. I was next up on the ladder when I heard him. My dad walks with the confidence of a colonel. The jangle of a pocket full of keys, coins, and golf tees got louder as each bold stride brought him closer. Between his teeth, he gripped the butt of a cigar, so his smile was crooked, the smile of a man who delights in mischief. He stood beside my mother and watched my budding ballerina legs climb the ladder, walk to the edge of the diving board, and jump, or in ballet terms *grand jeté*, into the sky.

I held freedom for as long as gravity would allow before plunging into the cool, deep water. The minute my head popped up to the surface, my dad barked through teeth that held the cigar: "Tara! What are you jumping for? That's for kids. I want you to dive."

I thought I qualified as a kid, but only replied, "I don't want to dive." Something told me this was not about what I wanted.

My dad snatched the cigar from his teeth. "Sure you do. You're going to dive. Get back up there and dive."

The sun was setting and my skin protested with little goose bumps as I climbed out of the pool. I was prepared to wait in line, knowing there was no way out. But the other kids had all backed away, waiting, watching. The lifeguards stopped cleaning, their eyes frozen on this scene. Twelve rungs stood between me and the plank. Shivering, I climbed the ladder and walked to the edge. My arms went up, perfectly aligned beside my ears. My toes gripped the board, my torso folded over and, with a small bend in the knees—or in ballet terms, *demi plié*—I prepared to dive. But as I pushed off, fear leaped in and with my body in a lopsided curve, I landed on my face and feet in one wet crash.

Humiliation burned off the goose bumps as I climbed out of the pool. I looked at the kids and young lifeguards, all staring at me. I bet they had fathers that they call Daddy—the cuddly kind of Daddy that puts his little girl on his shoulders, holding her closer to her dreams. I looked at my father and longed for him to be a Daddy. But my dad aimed to make his kids tough.

"Go again," he barked. "We aren't leaving until you dive."

My mom asked my dad to stop while my brothers started cheering for me to dive. I climbed the ladder, walked to the end of the plank, prepared to dive, and again, shaped like a confused candy cane, I crashed into the deep end.

From my chest down to my toes, I was burning. From the inside out, I felt a heat that, at nine years old, I didn't understand. Still, I knew that protesting would only make this worse. My mom tried again to deter my dad by insisting it was time to leave. I could also feel that my brothers were hurting with me. In desperation, they cheered me on, "C'mon Tara, dive! You can do it. Dive in!"

I ascended the ladder once more and right before my third attempt, I turned my head to look at my family—Mom's brows furrowed, eyes pleading. My brothers, tense and scared, continuing to shout encouragement that bordered on begging. They were helpless and only I could relieve their anguish. "Dive, Tara. You can do it. Dive." I wanted to ease their hurting, to love them back.

The burning turned to fuel. After another *demi plié*, I took to the air, my little ballerina legs pointing toward the sky, muscles taut from fingertips to pointed toes.

I landed in a perfect dive.

And yet, it would be the first and last time I ever dove off a platform higher than a swimmer's starting block.

On the way to the restaurant, I stared out the car window, teeth clamped tightly as I fought back tears. I recalled how the burning centralized in my gut and heart, turned into love, and shot me off that diving board. On that day, I made a promise to myself—never again would I let anyone make me feel as if a giant foot were pressed on my chest. Never again would anyone tell me there was only one way out. I wouldn't give anyone that power, the power to break me. For as long as I can remember, my mom told me, "Tara, you can do anything you put your mind to." Whether it was her words or a force that was born on a diving board, I have always felt an extra serving of fight in my belly. It's like a flame I can feel when I need to believe I can beat the odds. But truth is, I had no proof, because I had never really tested its power.

January 1996. For the past five years, I've stayed home with my kids, and kept other people's kids, to pay for the groceries I feed to the kids. I'm tired of being broke. I'm tired of wiping butts that weren't born to me. It's time to go out and talk to people who know how to blow their own nose.

My husband Billy and I agree, "It's time for a change." We're moving our young family of five from Atlanta to Watkinsville, Georgia, because I got a new sales job. Although I have a degree in journalism, my recent experience is in coupon clipping and creating stories that put toddlers to sleep. Nevertheless, I had talked my way into an interview I wasn't qualified for and, so I'm told, crushed the sales assessment. That's how I landed this job, that is not so much a job as it is buying a dream on credit. It is a chance to run my own business with the company paying a draw until I can operate in the black.

The thought of a new challenge and of wearing a bra to work excites me. From what I have ascertained, the potential for income is vast. The other sales reps in Georgia are a group of highly-driven, competitive white dudes who are amassing wealth at a rapid pace. Due to fierce competitors, I am taking on the only territory in the state that has never been profitable. My competition? Also, white dudes who make it their business to create deep, unbreakable bonds with their customers—high school principals. To win a sale in this business is to take the contract away from the competitor, deeming you the school's sole supplier for class rings, graduation invitations, caps and gowns, and diplomas.

During my first three years in this job, I learned to survive disappointment and failure on a grand scale. I studied every word, joke, strategy, and tactic of the successful men who coached me and cheered me on. My determination to win took over my rationale. Even as the other reps, one by one, suggested I do something else and that it wasn't my fault, I would not give up. The stress of a single-digit bank balance, a husband back in college to become a teacher, and three babies who insisted on eating every single day ignited my Hail Mary effort. I let go of trying to be one of the guys and created a path to winning that was in line with my heart for students and teachers. The scales started to tilt. The competitors stopped laughing at me. Then they criticized me. And then they tried to hire me.

I had my proof. The flame that was discovered on a diving board is the source of my fighting spirit. It's a little reservoir of fuel that I can tap into when a logical person would surrender. The losing, the disappointment, the naysayers—they all made my heart ache more than I ever admitted to anyone. But they never broke my spirit. I learned that the only person who has power over my spirit is me. What I didn't know is that I was going to need this truth for what was barreling toward me: the fight of my life.

CHAPTER 1

A LITTLE VIRUS

It's January 10, 2005, and I'm starting the five-hour drive home from a high school principals' convention in St. Simon's Island. I spent the past two and a half days attending meetings about graduation metrics, making memories on the golf course, and laughing late into the evenings with my expanding community of treasured customers. High school principals are some of the most passionate people on earth. My heart is full with gratitude for the career I am building. My mind shifts to home. I think of my family, and with the power of a freight train, the gratitude swells and pulses through me.

I call Billy from the car. He had taken our middle child Caroline to the pediatrician because she had a low-grade fever and a headache. The doctor told him it was just a little virus that would run its course.

Billy tells me he took Caroline back to the doctor because she has developed a rash all over her body. He says, "Dr. Fripp wasn't there, but Sherri (his nurse practitioner) called and asked him to come into the office because she thought the rash looked unusual. Dr. Fripp told Sherri that it's not uncommon for a little virus to cause a rash. She told us that he assured her Caroline would be fine and so we left."

"How is she?" I ask. "How is the fever?"

Billy tells me she is much better. The fever is gone, she is still a little tired, but she doesn't want to go back to school with the rash.

To a seventh grader, being at school with a rash does seem life-altering. "No problem," I say. "I'll stay home tomorrow with Caroline."

That evening after dinner, as the kids get ready for bed, I'm overcome with a sudden urge to hold my little girl. I dash upstairs, climb up into the tall, cherry, poster twin bed, gather her into my arms, and tell her, "I missed you so much while I was gone."

She snuggles in and laughs, "Well, I didn't miss you. Dad let me eat whatever I wanted."

I gently tickle her ribs to punish her for taking advantage of Dad's soft heart. Then she rolls to her side and tilts her head down toward her chest. She says nothing, but I know this cue. She used to ask, "Will you play with my under-hairs?" And I would gently stroke and smooth the hair at the base of her neck. She doesn't ask anymore, and it has been a long time since she cued me by exaggerating this position. I oblige and think how much I love being a mom. It lights my heart on fire.

The next morning, at about 9:30, I realize it's getting a bit late and I haven't heard a peep from Caroline. Oddly, a sense of panic ticks through me and I start running from the kitchen, up the stairs, and down the hall to her room. I walk over to where she lays, atop the tall canopy bed. She looks unnatural, her body contorted. I gently take her shoulder in my hand and shake it, whispering, "Caroline. Caroline."

And then louder, shaking her shoulder with real force, "Caroline! Wake up. Caroline!"

I stop shaking her and put my hands on either side of her face.

"Caroline, stop this! Caroline!" I insist, hoping it's a game.

I pull up one eyelid, let go, and watch it slip back over her eye. Now I'm screaming her name over and over.

I stare in horror as her eyes open and convulsions begin to ripple through my 12-year-old little girl. Her body jerks violently as her face turns blue. Her teeth rattle as her eyeballs roll almost out of sight and foamy saliva oozes from her clenched mouth.

My heart is banging madly inside my chest as my brain screams *911! Call 911!*

I have to find a phone, but if I leave her, she will fall off this damn bed. I take her torso and half lift, half drag her onto the carpet. I run again. Into my room. Out of my room.

"Where is a mobile phone?" I scream. "Downstairs! Shit!"

I run down, grab the phone and as my shaking hands dial 911, I torpedo back up the stairs. As I run down the hall and slide onto the floor beside Caroline, I see the convulsing has stopped. She is wet, motionless, completely limp.

"Yes, she is breathing." I tell the responders. "No, she has never had a seizure! Just hurry. Hurry." I hang up, call the school where Billy now works as a teacher, and ask the receptionist to send him home immediately. Minutes later, the responders arrive and rush a gurney into Caroline's room. She's breathing, but completely unresponsive. Billy's car screeches into the yard as they are loading her into the ambulance. Without waiting for permission, I climb in behind her and yell to Billy, "St. Mary's! Follow us."

He tries to ask me something, but the double doors close and we are moving. His car trails us as we speed the 10 miles from Watkinsville to Athens.

Caroline is rushed into the ER. We wait by her side as a lot of scrub-donned people inspect her with needles, tubes, and a variety of machines. Just as I trust the horror is over, the convulsing begins again. Her body is jerking like a machine gun. I can see every vein, every muscle, gang up to assault her delicate frame. From the blur of scrub-wearing people, we are told she needs to go to Atlanta. We're rushed into another ambulance, 65 miles of a siren blaring through traffic, and she is again rushed to the ER, this time inside Egleston Children's Hospital at Emory University.

My forehead is pressed into the cheap, white, over-bleached blanket. It feels harsh, yet dull. The monitor relentlessly beeps, communicating a sporadic, unsettling affirmation of life. It's been two and a half days and Caroline has only opened her eyes when the team of muscles unite to victimize her powerless body with violent convulsions.

My arm is hugging her long, lean legs. I'm begging. I'm begging God, "Please, please, let her wake up."

Saliva trickles and burns my throat as I plead through clenched teeth, "Come on Caroline, come back to me! I'm right here with you. Mom is here."

I try to will my fighting spirit directly into her heart. It's as though I can't get close enough; I want to melt into her.

"Please baby, please, open your eyes." I look up and even with the gauze and wires wrapped around her head and the tubes taped to her face, I see her petite, flawless profile. My mind is blurry black and purple. *This can't be real.* The maddening chirps of the monitors say otherwise.

Billy insists I take a break, so I peel myself away from my daughter's motionless body and leave the ICU in a trance. Wearing my ankle-length brown wool coat with the shimmery black lapels, I head outside. Standing in the icy wind, I glance to the ground and think how stupid I must look in aqua blue Nikes and this elegant coat. Reaching into the pocket, I pull out my best friend, a half-full box of Marlboro Lights and the mini pink lighter. A split second of pleasure teases me as I pull one slender cigarette from the box. I light the end, take a deep drag in, exhale, and let the security of the cigarette comfort me.

The cold against my face feels like a punishment I somehow deserve. It tells me to suffer, as if in solidarity with my child. I accept this bitter cold notion and use it to clear my head. Over the past few days, even the best disease specialists from the CDC have visited, investigated, and interrogated. They've got nothing.

I drop my glowing cigarette butt to the concrete and step on it with my Nike. After my last exhale of soothing smoke, I whisper into the cold, "Just a little virus, huh, Dr. Fripp?"

CHAPTER 2

PIMP HATS AND POISE

Sitting in the hospital, watching my daughter's lungs lift slightly off her heart and back down again, puts me in a trance. Frozen by shock and fear, I remain trapped, choking on the taste of helplessness. I can't take phone calls, I can't eat, I can't work or sleep. I can only think.

My mind goes back to eight months earlier. It was a belated birthday party because Caroline wanted to combine it with her best friend Catherine, making it also an end-of-sixth-grade dance party. They invited about sixty kids, picked out a bunch of junk food and, for some reason, they decided to buy hats. Matching pimp hats. Why pimp hats? I haven't a clue. But I must admit, they looked adorable in these wide brims, covered with fake zebra fur, hot pink trim and spunky feathers shooting up from the hatbands. I could almost hear the hats. They greeted you, saying, "Smile, life is now."

Pop music, laughter, and line-dances filled the gym, turning it into a sixth-grader's dream party. Each time a parent arrived to drop off their child, both seemed hesitant and a bit nervous about a party that had graduated from backyard games and goody bags. But before I could welcome them, something completely unexpected happened. Caroline turned into a host as if she had been in training with debutants. With poise and warmth, she extended her hand to every parent, introduced herself, and proceeded to share a little story about their child or a bit of admiration for how they added to her school experience. Caroline greeted people, checked on guests, and when she was sure everyone was feeling welcome, she joined in the dancing. I watched her embrace her friends with hugs and chatter. She laughed, animated, and even corralled the crowd for the Cha-Cha slide.

Of our three children, Caroline has always been the most reserved, never wanting the spotlight. Her older brother and younger sister both had dreams of trophies and stardom. Not Caroline. Since the fourth grade, she was clear and steadfast about her goals for the future. "I want to be a second-grade teacher. And I want to be a mom." That was all she asked for from this life. That night, we saw a 12-year-old aspiring teacher glide through a crowd with zero doubt as to where she was headed.

Billy and I were not the only ones in awe of her. Our daughter Holly was nine years old and completely enamored with her big sister. She joined in the dances and hung on every word as the girls giggled and gossiped. Whether talking to a 4-year-old or a 40-year-old, Holly dives into connection with the same uninhibited zeal. She knew many of the kids from swim team and cheerleading. So, she spent much of the night emulating dance moves or finding girls who would agree to practice cheerleading routines to the beat of Usher, Nelly, or Britney Spears. Every time I looked at Holly, I could see her contagious smile sparkle, filling her space with spirit.

Holly not only idolized Caroline, but she also completely adored her big brother. Wilson was born with some unique energy and an unquenchable curiosity. His body and mind never seemed to rest. He played soccer, football, and basketball with an innate drive and focus. Other than sports, Wilson was passionate about animals, the outdoors, and most of all, his social life. So as a 14-year-old rising freshman, he had no trouble surrounding himself with dance partners at Caroline's party. He danced with an easy playfulness and socialized with a charisma that flowed through his body. Although he spent the evening dancing and laughing with seventh-grade admirers, he took time to make one thing clear—he was the protector of Caroline and Holly.

As the night sped by, Billy and I glanced at each other. It was as if to say, "We're doing something right. Our kids are shining brightly; they are all healthy, confident, and happy."

I yearn to go back and savor those moments as the hospital monitors jolt me into reality.

After wiping my tears on the rough hospital blanket, I stand up, lean down, and cover Caroline's cheeks, her eyelids, her nose, and forehead with soft kisses. Maternal love clamps around my throat. My whole body wants to envelop her. Make her fully alive again. I want to go back and watch her one more time glide around that party and laugh with her friends.

The doctors won't commit to anything. "She has encephalitis," they explained. "The virus is causing inflammation in her brain. We are trying to reduce the swelling, but we can't be sure of the effects."

"She is going to wake up," I assure myself aloud. I know it. They don't know how much fight this little girl has in her. But I do. I sit back down, rest my chin on the bed, and smile, thinking about how she uses a resolute, almost methodical persistence to achieve what she sets her mind to.

Only a week ago, she was surrounded by a cheerleading squad that she had worked tirelessly to be a part of. To be frank, I am not a fan of cheerleading. Well, I love the performing and athleticism of the routines, I just hate the princess syndrome that comes with it. The dramatic makeup, the skimpy outfits, the booty shaking—these are not the priorities I want impressed on my daughters. Even still, I let Holly participate, and after the first cheer competition, Caroline came home determined not to remain a spectator in a seat beside her mother. Holly is a risk-taker by nature. She throws her entire body, mind, and spirit into all that she does. But Caroline is more cautious and analytical—not a natural athlete. Even so, she was determined. She started tumbling classes in hopes of earning a spot on one of these competition cheer squads. It felt like taking a lamb into a bull fight.

At 10 years old, Caroline learned through sheer will and guts. She ran to the mat, forcing her long legs to fly over her head and back down in time to fling her posture back-ward into a back handspring. She wasn't made to do this, but her mind rejected that notion. With piercing brown eyes and a hot red face framed by little dripping brown curls, she persevered.

The class would end, but she would not stop. Week after week, she kept trying, until finally she mastered this foundation for competition cheer: the round-off, back-hand spring. From there, it was like she believed she could do anything. She remained calm and resolute, and she kept getting better. She could do back handsprings over and over, spanning the length of the gym. With the same monomaniacal determination, she landed a back tuck. And with that, she earned a spot on the competition squad.

She *is* going to wake up. She has the spirit of a fighter.

CHAPTER 3
THE BULL

Through the tiny window shielded by cheap dusty blinds, a rising sun alerts me that another day has begun. Day 3. Throwing off the worthless hospital blanket, I will my weary body from the tiny daybed to kiss Caroline's forehead. In a melodic whisper, I feign the cheerful mom she has known:

"It's morning time. Time to wake up in the morning . . . and start your day."

I kiss her cheek, her fingers. No response.

I grab my duffle bag and head to the communal hospital shower and scrub and shave myself. I put on some sad mom jeans, an old purple sweater from the Gap, and my Nikes. I dry my hair and take 10 minutes to carefully apply makeup. Why put on makeup to spend the day in Caroline's hospital room?

I am motivated by the memory of a seven-year-old Caroline who once looked over at me in the car and said, "Mommy, you're pretty. But you're *more pretty* with makeup on." I threw my head back in laughter. My daughter was telling me I don't look too good in the raw. So today is the day I decide, I better look *more pretty* for Caroline when she wakes up.

A few hours later, I'm staring at Caroline, forcing myself to nibble an apple. Billy sits on the other side of her, wringing his hands and habitually wiping his forehead with his fingertips. It's silent, except for the torture of the monitors.

We both see it. Caroline opens her eyes. My heart races as I death-grip the apple and leap over to the bed, expecting another seizure. But this is different. Her eyes don't start to roll. She looks at my face. She looks at her dad. She looks back at me, her eyes filled with terror. And then, she starts screaming.

"Who are you? Where's my mom? I want my mom. Get away! You have an apple coming out of your face!"

She tries to sit up, but is restrained by wires and tubes. She rips at the IV in her arm and the wires on her head, unable to make sense of her surroundings. The scrub team runs in and holds her arms and legs as she fights to escape the bed.

"Get off me! Leave me alone! Get off!" she screams in terror.

Someone runs in with straps and works to Velcro my daughter to the bed.

This horror show goes on repeat, interrupted only by shots of Ativan and Xanax from the scrub team. For two more days, it's seizures, outbursts, drugs, restraints.

Everyone keeps telling me to leave her side. Get out. Walk. Eat. I oblige mindlessly, but only long enough to consume caffeine or nicotine, and then return like a puppet with no will of its own. The pain in my gut feels like a raging bull. The longer I contain him, the angrier he gets.

On Day 5, a nurse tells me it's time for a break; we have visitors, but they aren't permitted into the ICU. As I enter the waiting room, I see two of Caroline's best friends from school and their mothers, who have driven all the way to Atlanta to show their devotion. A rational mind would have run to them with gratitude, accepting hugs of comfort and support. I was not functioning with a rational mind.

The familiarity of the two innocent faces scorches me without warning. From my gut, the raging bull breaks free.

I scream out across a waiting room packed with anxious, emotional people, "Get those kids out of here!" I heave in a sob so massive it expands my entire chest. I crumple over and wail, trying to rid my body of the agony. Someone grabs me and gently helps me stand and walk away.

My behavior shocks even me. What the hell happened? I tell myself I snapped because I was protecting my daughter from friends seeing her in this exorcism-like state. But they don't even let visitors in the ICU, I remember. The most honest part of me knows what really spewed out of me. Jealousy. *I'm jealous.* I want it to be *my* seventh grader standing there in low-rise blue jeans and frosty pink lip gloss. I ache for my daughter to be like these kids—kids who recognize their mom, kids who are going to gossip between classes tomorrow and make plans for the weekend.

With this bitter taste of self-awareness, I compose myself and apologize. But to this day, I can see their little faces, eyes frozen open when I exploded like a bull from his chute.

The hospital room is equipped with video and sound recording devices. They help the neurologists review and study seizures. So, every moment of this nightmare is being captured on camera. Billy and I are sitting on either side of Caroline when the phone rings again. Friends, family, and colleagues keep calling with prayers, offers to help, and expressions of support, hope, and love. Thankfully, Billy has taken the role of receptionist.

He answers, speaks a minute, and says to me, "It's Connie Martin. Says her daughter and Caroline are friends. She wants to check on you."

I think, *that's kinda weird. I don't really know her.*

I had let Caroline go over to her house a few times where they gathered in the yard with a large group of other middle school kids. Caroline had told me that the boys laugh at Connie Martin because she has a habit of leaning out of the upstairs window to check on the kids. All the boys snicker because she doesn't just pop her head through the open window; she leans her entire torso out over the ledge, showing off a fluffy new boob job.

This image pops in my head as Billy hands me the phone. "Tara. This is Connie Martin, Hayleigh's mom. I wanted to call and say I'm sorry and I'm praying for Caroline." I thank her and then she says, "One more thing. Is whatever Caroline has contagious?"

Silence. I cannot speak as the bull starts to rage inside my gut. To fill the silence, she continues, "Caroline was at our house just a few days before y'all went to the hospital. So, I'm worried about my girls. I'm sorry to ask, but what does she have? Are we at risk?"

Although I'm stunned, I speak with emotionless pragmatism, "No Connie. The doctor told us it was just a little virus. But Caroline now has encephalitis, which is not contagious. So you can just go on about your life. You don't need to worry about your girls. I sure hope I have made you feel better."

She stammers. I hang up.

The bull breaks free. "Can you believe the self-serving nerve of that woman, Billy? She did not call to check on me or Caroline. She called to see if Caroline is *contagious*! How sick is that? What a conniving bitch! The next time I see her, I won't be able to control myself. I'm going to take those fake tits and wrap them around her neck!"

"Tara!" Billy jerks his thumb up and down, pointing at the camera facing me. "Be quiet!"

My mouth is poised to continue my rant, but I stop. I look up at the camera, then at Billy.

We burst out laughing. For several minutes, we can't stop. The release of endorphins is euphoric. For a moment, it's just us again, laughing within our trusted bond and unfiltered commentary.

CHAPTER 4
A PASTOR AND A BONG SONG

It's Day 7 in the ICU. Caroline wakes up and I brace myself for either a seizure or another scene of confusion, terror, and thrashing. But no seizure. No rage. She blinks and slightly furrows her brow. She tries to grab the feeding tube, but the Velcro keeps her wrists cuffed to the bed rails. I rip off one of the straps, hold her dry hand, and search her eyes.

"Mom?" she whispers. "Am I in the hospital?"

I hear Billy behind me. He has this way of trying to hold back tears that results in a choke and chuckle. The familiar sound pierces my heart as gratitude and relief wash over me.

Caroline is stabilizing; the seizures are less frequent and shorter. The scrub team moved her into a regular room where she will start intensive therapy. Here she can have visitors—and I can have emotional outbursts that will not be recorded. I'm losing track of the days, of life outside these pale-yellow walls. I think I should be doing something, but I don't know what. In response to Caroline, I jump into action. But outside of that, even getting up to get myself a cup of water takes some convincing inside my head.

As the days tick by, I try to process what we know. The brain is complex, the most studied and the least understood organ in the human body. Caroline's diagnosis is traumatic brain injury (TBI), caused by encephalitis from a virus of unknown etiology. The secondary diagnosis is seizure disorder, also caused by encephalitis. The neurologists explained that no two TBI cases are alike.

Caroline has gone from a coma, to scenes from a horror movie, to now. She sleeps no more than 45 minutes per day for the next 12 days. She can't eat or swallow, she can't write, sit up on her own, walk, or even hold her hairbrush. But boy, can she talk. The TBI has damaged the part of her prefrontal cortex where the brain's filter is housed, the part that prevents us from verbalizing every unedited thought. Caroline talks incessantly and without this filter, she blurts out every thought as if she is on a quest to break the world's record for longest soliloquy. She is loud, inappropriate, a little rude, and comical, keeping every visitor and clinician laughing. Billy and I are also laughing, but as a release. We are relieved— she is going to live. It is all that matters in this moment.

Caroline welcomes every visitor the same way, which is completely devoid of the Caroline she was only two weeks ago. Doctors, nurses, therapists, friends, and night sitters are all greeted with the chorus of "Colt 45 and Two

Zigzags" by Afroman. Covered in electrodes and wrapped in gauze, her little head bops as she finishes with, "And smoke that tumbleweed."

It was funny the first, oh, 20 times or so. But I start to think, *really now? You don't remember how to brush your teeth or hold a spoon, yet these gangster lyrics are flawlessly stored in your mind?* My delirium just lets it be. When our pastor is greeted with an invitation to hit a bong like Cheech and Chong, all I can do is feign a little shock.

The doctors assure us Caroline is out of danger and on the mend, so tonight Billy's father will drive Wilson to the hospital for a visit. It's only around 8:00 a.m., so I decide to race home, reload my overnight bag, and get back in time to see my son. I believe I will tap into some renewed energy if I can just breathe outside of fluorescent lights and the smell of sanitizers, hear a bird chirp rather than a monitor, and most of all, see Holly.

I drive to Watkinsville and straight into the elementary school parking lot. As I speed-walk up the corridor to the entrance, I think back to our last parent-teacher conference. Miss Spalding had assessed our fourth-grader by saying, "Holly is whip smart. Also, she is highly sensitive and intuitive. Her motivation and her propensity to worry are both off the charts. Holly will be one of two things. She will be amazing. Or she will be a mess. There is no middle ground for her."

"Amazing. Definitely amazing," I mutter to myself as I approach all the smiling women in the front office. They gush and hug and tell me about all the churches that have Caroline on their prayer lists. I envy their essence, like cupcakes, light and sweet. But I am in a war. I'm barred from sweetness. They ask for information, but I stick to my mission:

"I just need to check Holly out for the day, please."

I sign the clipboard's ledger and race down the hallway to Miss Spalding's room. Desperate to inhale the love that emits from this kid, I open the classroom door and my eyes find Holly. She is all in, fully devoted to her worksheet. With intensity wrapped around her pencil, she is sitting on her foot folded under her, quickly filling in answers.

Miss Spalding sees me in the doorway and softly calls out, "Holleee." Holly's head pops up and she sees me. "Mommy!" Her chair tumbles backward as she runs into my arms.

No one can hug like Holly Pauline. No hesitation, no caution, no partial commitment. Miss Spalding's assessment rings in my mind: "There is no middle ground for Holly."

Thank God, I say to myself, as I hold my baby and drink in her spirit.

The short trip to see Holly helped me to recharge. As I walk back into Caroline's hospital room, I'm reminded that she has come a long way from a coma and then a state of complete amnesia. Even though she is not the sensitive, quiet girl she was, there is still reason to celebrate. At least we think so—until her brother arrives. Wilson's grandfather walks him into the hospital room. I grab him, smother him with kisses, and breathe him in. As my eyes close, I can smell my old life—energy, laughter, and our Boxer, Bruiser. I smell cleats, Zaxby's, and a backpack filled with textbooks, notebook paper, and #2 pencils.

Wilson's pencils are not only for school; he plays them. Yep, he plays the pencils. With one in each hand, adding in knuckles and palm for bass and effects, Wilson can play the pencils using the kitchen counter as the drum. With speed and adrenaline, he keeps a giant smile while beating out one rhythm after the next.

As I treasure this memory, I pull back and look into my son's face, a hollow version of the one that I know. He turns away to greet his sister.

"Wilson! Wilson, I've been missing you," Caroline squeals. "Wilson, I know you gave me my nickname Cabooh when I was a baby, but I have a new nickname. Look at my head; I am Wire Woman. These people keep asking me a lot of questions, like what day it is. Don't they know what day it is? I have a screwed-up brain now, so why are they asking me what day it is and who the president is? They are the doctors. Shouldn't they know who George Bush is?"

Wire Woman chats on as I watch my son try to keep smiling. But he can't. Tears glisten in his topaz-blue eyes. His lower lip trembles as he looks over at me. Before we can comfort him, Wilson runs. I run after him, grab his sweatshirt, and pull him to me. But he fights me off.

"Why is everyone so happy? That's not my sister. Why is she acting like that?" He chokes on a sob. "That's not my sister!"

@

Another week passes and it is finally time to leave Egleston Children's Hospital. Wilson and Holly have been at home with my mother for more than three weeks. When I call home, Holly usually answers. Sentiments pour out: "Mom! When are you coming home? Grandma is crying all the time. Wilson is never here. I hate it here."

Finally, I'm able to tell her, "Soon, Honey. We are coming home tomorrow. Caroline is very different, though. She repeats herself a lot and she makes odd jokes. Everyday though, she gets just a little bit better. The doctors say she will keep getting better, back to how she used to be."

The day has come. No more Wire Woman, just a little glue residue left in Caroline's baby-fine, oak-colored hair, which she can now brush herself. She's wobbly, but she can walk. Dressed in her royal blue and black cheerleading warm-up suit, she's ready to go, except for her shoes. I hand her a sneaker, holding my breath. *Please remember, remember how to tie shoes.*

She does! It takes some time and concentration, but it's one down, one to go. And then she moans, her hand and leg stiffen, and her dad grabs her before the seizure can cause her to hit the floor. Billy holds onto her, and I ring for a nurse. When she finally goes limp and begins breathing again, I smell something. It's urine. She is covered in urine. I think about the middle school cool-kid crowd anxiously awaiting Caroline's return. Cool kids can be mean kids, and very discriminating about who is allowed to remain in their circle. Will they unite and push Caroline out of their exclusive posse? I think of Wilson and Holly. How will Wilson feel to see a sister he has lived to protect, wet herself? How will Holly react to see a sister she idolizes lose her decorum to convulsions?

CHAPTER 5
LORETTA

It has been more than nine years since I took the job that gave me a snowball's chance in hell of growing a business. And now, the business is growing and thriving. Rather than continuing to try and fit a mold, to emulate my competitors, I created a brand of my own. I learned to do something different—to be in service to students and teachers. I contributed to achievement by creating leadership workshops and reward programs for students and by giving inspirational talks at assemblies and faculty meetings.

And those dudes on my team, the ones with the giant egos? Well, it turns out, they have hearts to match. They have become my brothers. I never even asked; they simply stepped up to take care of my business. Also, within the high schools I serve, I have built deep, trusting friendships. Thanks to the support of my colleagues and clients, Billy can keep teaching while I focus on Caroline's rehabilitation. For the next 10 weeks, Monday through Friday, I drive her 65 miles each way to a center for brain injury patients in Atlanta.

On the first day, we walk up to a window where no one is in sight. Caroline peers through the glass and begins to bang on the counter, yelling, "Hello! I'm Caroline. Wire Woman is here! My brain is screwed up. I'm here so you can fix it!"

Bright pink scrubs, wiry black hair, and a smile framed by deep dimples greet us: "Hi Caroline. I'm Loretta. We are so glad you're here." Loretta signs us in and walks us back to a large communal area.

The room is filled with bobbing heads and twisted facial expressions. It pulsates with moans, yelps, and odd-sounding laughs. Wheelchairs, helmets, drool, indiscernible words, and blank stares flood my senses. I blink hard and think back to the hundreds of times I had thanked God for my blossoming children, never stopping to consider I could be a mom with anything but. Imagining their families fills me with a new depth of compassion.

The kids who came to visit Caroline in the hospital appear in my mind and again that surge of jealousy prickles my skin. I see their moms' faces too, and how they looked at me. With their brows deeply furrowed, I could feel their yearning to ease the unimaginable. I could feel their desperation, because four short weeks ago, I was one of them, a mom with children who scored above-average development at the pediatrician's office. And now?

Could I be a mother of a special needs child? I realize how shallow my gratitude has been. I never stopped to consider how it might feel to raise a child who will need significant and unique support. Never again will I encounter someone with exceptional challenges and be able to dismiss the extraordinary effort that goes into managing what I used to take for granted as the basics of daily life. These thoughts dust me with shame.

I try to shake off the nagging revelation by returning my focus to my daughter. She is lockstep with Loretta as we take a tour of this haven for TBI patients. The tour was quick, too quick. It's time for me to leave Caroline here for the day. My stomach roils like a sea of curdled milk.

As if I own the room, I announce to the staff, "You understand she has seizures. She could crash down at any minute. She needs to be in soft surroundings."

They stare.

I continue. "She can't be on stairs or ledges or near hot surfaces, and—"

They assure me they've got this. I thank them. They wait. I wait. They nod toward the door. I start to go. I turn back. Loretta brings her dimples up toward the corners of her knowing eyes, puts her arm around me, and guides me out.

A vaguely familiar emotion seeps in. What is it? Oh, yes. It's the feeling I had the first time I parted with Wilson as a newborn. I was going to get my haircut, for God's sake. He was six weeks old and as I handed him over to my sweet mother-in-law, it felt like I was leaving one of my limbs in her arms. I couldn't fathom not being able to hold him, to kiss him, to protect him, and to make him smile.

As I dart from the TBI center to the parking deck, I'm reminded of the promises I made to myself when I was pregnant for the first time. Unlike my childhood home, I was intent on creating a home that pulsed with joy. We would play games, crank up music, dance, and break a few rules. Before this war on seizures and brain injury, cooking dinner very often included blaring Van Morrison from the CD player. I would dance the Carolina Shag with Wilson and then Holly, delighted in the moment as I spun her around. Caroline prefers to watch this silliness, but sometimes I could twirl her a bit, too. And when their dad busted out his impressive dance moves, it was pure joy.

Pulling my car out of the parking deck, I yearn for a moment back in the kitchen where worries are put on hold and smiles dance like sunlight on the river. I become desperate for my secret savior, the Marlboro Lights. My hands fumble for the pack and light a cigarette as I zoom away. My cheeks are pinned into my jaw, I can't get air past the tip of my lungs, and I don't know where I'm going.

I pull into the first random parking lot I see and try to finish the cigarette, but all I can think about is finding glass. Glass vases. Big, heavy, glass vases. I need them so I can throw them at a brick wall—the side of our red brick house will do. I imagine an industrial-sized bucket filled with vases that I am smashing, one by one, against our house.

And I see something more. I see a face; it's a face to blame. I see Caroline's pediatrician, Dr. Fripp. He had called the hospital countless times, but I wouldn't speak to him. He had been too busy to come and see the rash that his nurse practitioner was worried about. If he had come that day, I was convinced, he would have administered steroids and Caroline would be in Social Studies right now with her friends. A rhythmic chant accompanies the vision of hurling glass at our brick home. On loop, it booms inside my head.

This is all your fault, Dr. Fripp. All your fault. All your fault.

I realize I've been gripping the steering wheel as if I can rip it loose, when my head slumps forward and I stop fighting off the pain. A foreign sound escapes my throat as my torso heaves. I let go of the wheel, of the past, and say goodbye to what my life looked like only weeks ago.

Hope gives me strength—not the kind of hope that is gift-wrapped in some irrational belief in miracles. When it's tied to action or facts, it becomes attainable, and hope fortifies me. Remembering the neurologists' predictions is a reason for hope. They all agreed that the healing would be rapid at first, but then it would slow. We were to trust that it will continue, even though it will be slight, barely noticeable.

We begged them for a prognosis. They were cautious and apologetically told us there is no way to predict. But one old neurologist, with little, round, wire glasses and a classic St. Nick beard saw the desperation in our eyes and pulled Billy and me into a little huddle.

In a deep, comforting voice, he said, "Look, if I were a betting man, I would say she's going to be just fine. Maybe a slight learning disability, but other than that, I'm betting she will be just fine."

Ten weeks later, I'm still trusting in St. Nick's prediction as I walk into the rehab center for the last time. They are having a graduation ceremony where the patients each wear a cap and gown that would have been rejected by Goodwill. The patients are presented with a certificate documenting attendance. The first little graduate I see is one I will never forget. Five-year-old Jack has his graduation cap duct-taped to the protective helmet he wears. With adventure-seeking eyes and a confident grin, Jack greets everyone in the room, again and again.

I had already met Jack's parents, who wear shirts and ball caps that say, "You don't know Jack." A year and a half ago, a smart, energetic three-year-old Jack and his family were out on a boat on Georgia's Lake Lanier. Jack fell out of the boat and the propeller sliced his head open. The doctors didn't expect him to live and if he did, they said, he probably wouldn't have enough cognitive function to communicate, walk, or learn. A single boat ride has rewritten Jack's entire life trajectory. Yet his parents are glowing with relief and victory. Their little boy is walking around the center, forming words, smiling like a college kid on spring break.

Jack and his family transformed my understanding of suffering on this earth. It comes at you from an untapped depth of darkness and abolishes what you thought mattered forever. Amid the suffering, even the slightest bit of light brings a burst of gratitude powerful enough to knock you to your knees. Like mirror balls dancing in darkness, Jack's parents are rejoicing.

Only a few months ago, I could not have comprehended this. But today, I get it. Nothing is more precious than this minute in time. The finality of yesterday's horror and the threat of tomorrow's anguish do not inhibit Jack's parents from diving headfirst into right here and now.

When the graduation reception of Chips Ahoy and Hawaiian Punch is over, it's time to say goodbye. Loretta holds Caroline and with tears in her eyes and a trembling voice, she says, "Caroline, when you go back to school, you will feel like a star. Honey, you just remember this will wear off. The ones who are still there are your real friends. The rest of them aren't worth worrying about."

She releases Caroline and hands her an envelope. "I wrote you a poem, Wire Woman. You keep it and whenever you're having a bad day, take it out and read it. Remember, Loretta loves you."

Loretta's wisdom travels with me to this day.

CAROLINE

No words will ever really describe the girl we all know as simply Caroline,
But there's nothing simple about her at least not in my mind.
It all started with a knock, knock is anybody there as she entered the place,
And from that moment on we knew we'd never forget her smiling face.

Each day she entered with a smile and we were glad to see her come,
Just as we were sad when she had to leave, once the day was done.
Caroline you have a special way of making things go right,
Even when it looks like, there's no hope in sight.

The smaller kids look up to you, as you encourage them to fight,
And taught them losing isn't bad if you played the game just right.
Follow the rules and do your best is what I heard you say,
And then you'd smile and hold their hand as they continue to play.

Now these words you use to calm the kids down each day,
I want you to remember that they apply to you in a way.
As you go back to school and reenter your old world again,
Nothing has change within your heart and return with a grin.

For your smile speaks a million words and will take you very far,
So return to school and take your place as a little superstar.
Your fame will be brief once they figure out that you're the same old girl,
And those who turn away from you never belonged in your world.

So remember it's the person that makes a name, Caroline,
And yours is world famous already and also well defined.
Know that, everyone will miss you, especially me each day,
But never forgotten in our hearts, we include you as we pray.

(A poem from the heart, maybe not well written but filled with love)
I'll miss you.
Loretta

CHAPTER 6
A YOO-HOO AND A MOON PIE

Spring break is over and it's time to return to school. Caroline, two months out of her TBI therapy, is excited. I'm a wreck. Without question, she will have a seizure at school at some point. And I know two things: first, I can't protect her forever and, second, I have a business to run.

Billy and I don't want Caroline to ride the bus, so I arrange my schedule to drop her off at the middle school and proceed to work, where I inspire students from a stage or sell them keepsakes that celebrate their achievements. I can feel the irony traveling up my spine.

Driving away from Oconee County Middle School on this first day, my chest feels as if a balloon is expanding inside it. When it reaches the point of pain, I realize I'm not breathing and let out a loud gush of air. But the tightness remains. As I grip the steering wheel, my throat swells and my ears grow hot before I let myself sob. I wonder how, at 39 years old, I never really knew what it felt like to cry. Driving south on Highway 15, I want to rid myself of this heartache by projecting it onto something or someone else. Through clenched teeth, I mutter what has been on repeat inside my head: *"This is your fault, Dr. Fripp. Since you couldn't be bothered with Caroline's rash, I just witnessed my once lively, engaging daughter walk into school heavily sedated, wrought with insecurities, hoping to resurrect a life she once had."*

I snatch my Jittery Joe's coffee from the cupholder, take a swig, fire up a Marlboro Light, and continue racing down the country highway. I have always loved the solitude on the road—just me, my coffee, my cigarettes, and my thoughts. My thoughts used to be oriented toward planning speeches, sales strategies, kids' schedules, and social events, but today I think about the past few months.

Our genuine, loving pastor Pam has been steadfast. She came to the hospital many times, and then to our home to listen and to pray with us. I think of all the people who tell me they are praying for us and that they put Caroline on their church's prayer list. Many of these folks give me the same encouraging comment, "Everything happens for a reason." I used to believe this and would have said the same to someone in my position.

But I now see it as trash talk. Every time I hear someone say *everything happens for a reason*, anger gurgles inside me. There is no way what has happened to Caroline is a loving God's will. If God is using my daughter to make other people feel gratitude, or whatever the hell, I can't accept that. No. No way, God. This cannot be your idea, your perfect plan. Just as I can't believe your playbook calls for torture, rape, abuse, or any other insidious suffering, a loving God can't be behind this horror my family is living.

But I do believe in something, something that grows more powerful with each passing day. I believe it is our responsibility to bring good from tragedy. I promise myself, I promise my family, that this inconceivable pain will not be for nothing. From our suffering, I will deliver something into this world that matters. But the first promise is to Caroline. With the universe, any and all gods, my car and this highway as my witnesses, I promise her, *Hang in there, baby. I am your warrior. I will find a way to stop these seizures and give you your life back.*

The flame that I discovered on a diving board at nine years old fuels me today. I will stop at nothing. No therapy, no surgery, no diet will be left unexplored. No option is off the table. I will find a way.

Too many times to count, I find myself speeding back to the middle school because Caroline has had a seizure. I abruptly leave a sales meeting or call one of my accounts to ask for forgiveness because I won't make it. Today the school nurse calls and says, "Caroline had a seizure. She's in the clinic and we changed her clothes. She has a bump on her head, but she's okay."

The nurse, a mischievous, loyal, lover of life named Kathleen, is the best friend you wish you had, but you can't have her. She's mine. I screech into the parking lot, leap out of the Explorer and run right past the front office to her clinic. When I hear Caroline's giggle, I stop outside the door and listen. Kathleen is telling Caroline:

"Girl, you have it made. This whole school is revolving around you. No one is laughing at you. They wish they *were* you! You're in here eating purple grapes with me, and they're sitting in Algebra, listening to Mr. Franks try to explain formulas. Oh, and hey, when your mom gets here, tell her I gave you a Yoo-hoo and a Moon Pie for lunch. Then we can watch her twitch."

I peek in and see Caroline laughing at Kathleen's she-nanigans. "Moon Pies!" I belt out. With that, I try to hold back tears as I grip-hug Kathleen.

As we help Caroline get ready to go home, my eyes lock into Kathleen's and I whisper, "You know we are going to beat this, right? It's not permanent."

"All I know," Kathleen replies, "is that if I ever get sick, I want you in charge."

Not accepting circumstances seems to be a pattern in my life. At 17 years old, I graduated from high school in Irmo, South Carolina. I wanted to move to New York to train to be a professional ballerina. My mom insisted that I start in Atlanta and go to college as well. So I went to Georgia State University in the mornings and trained at the studio the rest of the day.

After that year, I no longer wanted the life of a dancer, but I had fallen in love with city life, new friends, and the diversity at GSU. My dad said if I quit dancing and wanted to stay in school, I would have to come home and go to the University of South Carolina, where he could pay in-state tuition. Because of his salary, I couldn't qualify for support, and I couldn't qualify for a loan without a parent's signature.

Never again will anyone tell me that I only have one option, I reminded myself.

When I inquired about resident's status, the admissions counselor told me that a full-time job would qualify me. He explained that I would have to stop school for a year or just take a few classes, because I couldn't work full-time and stay in school full-time. He said, "It would be too tough. That's not an option. You will have to delay your four-year plan."

The familiar burning centralized in my gut and I thought, *Watch me.* I took a 7:50 a.m. class, worked all day at an insurance agency, and took night classes four days a week for a full year. In the spring of my fourth year in Atlanta, in accordance with my plan, I graduated.

Many years later, while I was busting my ass and failing at my sales job, colleagues tried to console me. They said I was put into a territory with impenetrable competitors, and that I was trying to achieve the impossible. The word *impossible* is gasoline to my flame.

Now it's 2005 and I am on a relentless quest to restore Caroline's life. With every seizure, hope waivers, it scratches at the back of my neck to suggest I can't complete the mission. The burning in my gut fights back and I think, *Watch me.* I will not stop until we give these seizures the big final *fuck you.* Caroline will heal and live out her plan to become a second-grade teacher and a mom.

As long as I keep working toward the win, I keep hope alive. I can't have hope without action, and to lose hope would smother me. Knowing this, I suspect I'm using this win-at-all-costs mentality to survive. But it comes with a price. My children need me to sit with them, to hold them, to let them feel my strength *and* my softness.

But I'm afraid, afraid to stop running and feel not only my grief, but my children's wounds, wounds that are raw and foreign to them. They were a pack of three active, lively, bickering kiddos. Now they face a journey for which they are totally unequipped. It was instilled in me as a child that to slow down or to be without a goal in sight is a weakness. But now, I see slowing down and cradling pain as something I am simply not strong enough to do.

CHAPTER 7

SWIMMERS TAKE YOUR MARKS

As the spring turns toward summer, I sign up all three kids for swim team, just as I have for many years. I'm sitting at the kitchen counter talking about swimsuit sizes and practice schedules with Holly.

She asks me, "Are you sure Caroline should swim this year? I mean, won't that be—"

A faint moan shoots me off the kitchen stool.

I run into the study.

"Caroline!"

I'm too late. She has flipped the chair over and is seizing under it.

"Holly, help me! I'll get the chair off her. Hold her head so it stops hitting the desk."

Ten-year-old Holly holds onto her big sister's head, putting her little hand between it and the wooden desk. With each violent jerk, Holly's knuckles take the hit.

When the jerking finally stops, I nestle onto the floor with Caroline, softly blowing cool air onto her face and kissing her gently. Holly carefully rests Caroline's head down on the carpet, steps over her limp body, and climbs the stairs, two at a time.

Holly never finished that sentence, but I know what she was going to say. The tension that frames her once-ebullient face said it first—she is afraid, for herself and for Caroline. But she doesn't dare mention her own angst, because it will be dismissed with the inferred or spoken retort that it pales in comparison to her sister's. She was going to express a fear that has suddenly barred us from living fully. Holly and I used to open our hearts to the world, welcoming perspectives and ideas as an invitation to engage. But now, we live trapped in a cautious, frantic state, witnessing other people living their carefree moments.

Just a few days ago, I exited Publix with my groceries. It was about 90 degrees without a cloud in the sky as Caroline and I walked across the steaming hot parking lot. Heat increases the chance of a seizure, so I moved quickly and kept thinking, *We are almost there. Just get her off this pavement and into the car.*

We made it. She got in the front seat. I steadied the cart against the curb and raced around the Explorer to crank the engine and turn on the air. As I loaded the bags into the hatch, a man called to me from a few cars away, "Your kid just sits in the car while you load the groceries?"

My heart rate increased, but my mouth wouldn't open. He stared at me, opening his hands as if to receive a response, then dropped his arms, and shook his head in frustration. I wanted to shove my cart right into his knees. But instead, as if to apologize for my poor parenting, I glanced back timidly like a scolded child. Inside the vehicle, I studied my face in the mirror and wondered, *Who is this cowering woman?*

❦

About half of encephalitis patients don't survive the onset of the condition. Because Caroline survived, Billy and I agree, even when there is risk, we must help Caroline live life to her capacity. What life would she have if we kept her crying on the sidelines? And so, despite our 10-year-old's warning, Caroline is back on the swim team this summer.

Wilson's swimming ability is probably average, but it's his intense desire to win that keeps him earning ribbons. In years past, I would watch him and think, *I get you, my son. You keep going after life with that kind of grit. Don't ever let anyone or anything break your fighting spirit.* But now, I see that his fight to win is also an escape, a race away from the emotional suffering. Yes, I do see the apple and tree analogy here.

This summer, Wilson's competitive drive is on overload. His home, once a safe haven, is racked with anxiety, heartache, and a sister who may never return to the one he always knew. Now, when Wilson loses a race, he loses control. He fights to turn tears into a tough anger. I watch a 15-year-old boy berate himself for a less than stellar performance.

"I slipped a little on the block. And then—" he tries to continue as his strong chest heaves. "I screwed up my turn. But I can beat those guys. I have beat them so many times!"

He throws his treasured silver swimming goggles into the fence and swats away my attempts to comfort him.

Unlike Wilson, Holly is about as competitive as a starfish. Even so, this is the sport that Holly excels in more than tumbling and cheerleading. Her little, strong body powers down the swim lane as if she were built for the water. She swims breaststroke and butterfly primarily. But she also swims the Individual Medley (one lap each of all four strokes), because the coach wants the win. Her coach gets so excited watching her, "Go Holly! Pull! Stop smiling and swim!"

Once, the coach looked at me as Holly effortlessly took the lead and said, "Mrs. Heaton, look at Holly. Not only is she still smiling, she is *chewing gum!*" He threw up his hands, shook his head with a quizzical grin and continued to pace the concrete with his clipboard.

Almost from birth, Holly seemed to hug life with a full-blown smile, limitless energy, and an inquisitive mind. At regional swim meets, she broke two state records. Billy and I saw college scholarships. But Holly insists she doesn't really like swimming. Being on the team is fun, but, says the smiling little starfish, "I don't really like the races."

Swim meets used to feel like the pinnacle of joy for a parent. In summers past, there was no need for excessive safety, no hiding my trauma, no feigning happiness. I just dove right into the joy of watching my kids not only compete, but cheer for each other. There was nothing to fake and nothing to fear.

But this summer, the summer of 2005, that changed

forever. At the pool, there is no safe space for Caroline. Would she have a seizure in the water? It would be silent. No one would hear. Everyone is already splashing and jerking about in the pool; maybe no one would even notice. And so, as I try to talk to other moms and give Wilson and Holly the attention they deserve, my eyes are glued to Caroline.

It's her first meet of the season. Backstroke was her specialty. From the time she was eight years old, she could glide across the water with a smooth, graceful rotation.

She's in the water, at the start. We hear from the loudspeaker, "Swimmers take your marks!" Just like the other swimmers, she pulls herself up and forward, gripping the starting block. The gun sounds and she's off. Watching her glide, Billy and I are frozen, tears spilling onto our cheeks.

She isn't fast anymore, but the fluid precision of her strokes is the same. Slowly, methodically, Caroline is backstroking her way to the finish line. Lane six, last place. As the other five swimmers finish, the cheering doesn't die down, it becomes louder. It pulses through our bodies. I feel the roar under my feet as I glance up to take in the surroundings.

Everyone is cheering for Caroline—both coaches, all the swimmers from both teams, and all the parents are rooting for her: "Go Caroline! Go! We love you, Caroline!"

My throat swells and my heart leaps with gratitude. When she finally finishes, Wilson is there, proudly helping her out of the pool. "Way to go, Caroline! You should be really proud of yourself," he says as he pulls a towel around her and escorts her through the crowd like a lion with his

45

cub. In this moment, I feel assured that Billy and I have made the right decision to let Caroline live life as a participant rather than a spectator.

The reassurance was short-lived. By about the third swim meet of the season, we realize it is too much on her. She can't handle the practices and, hell, neither can I. We ask if she would consider trying again next year, and with serious contemplation, she agrees. But she still wants to go to the meets, cheer on her brother and sister and be with her friends. As much as I imagine that would feel like throwing chlorine in a wound, I agree.

It's one of the last meets of the summer. Overdrive is my new heartrate. My nerves are fried crispy. The heat mixed with constant stress and fear brings about the kind of exhaustion that makes you beg for your bed. My mind keeps seeing all the times Caroline has crashed down with no warning. I smile and pretend to see people, but I can't see past my fear.

I follow Caroline around like a jealous boyfriend until, like any teenager would, she finally snaps and tells me, "This is pissing me off." She tries to assure me, "Mom, my friends are here. If I have a seizure, they've got it."

No, they haven't "got it," but I realize I must find a way to loosen my tension and let this community help protect Caroline. *Her life was not spared to keep her from living.* And so, I back off. I try to look at Holly when she talks to me. I try to cheer Wilson on while I watch him swim.

I wonder if it might be okay for me to sit down. I decide, maybe just for five minutes, and slowly ease myself into a lounge chair. I stare at my two tanned calves stretched out in front of me, swollen from standing in this humidity. I let out a gush of oxygen and think, *yes, this sitting down gig is a winner.*

A big crowd is forming at the other end of the pool, and Caroline has disappeared into it. Dammit. Why can't those kids just get the hell out of the way so I can see my baby? The crowd is getting bigger and at the same time, some kids are running toward me. The frantic little Speedo children are yelling.

"Mrs. Heaton! It's Caroline! She's having a seizure!"

Fuuuuuuuck, my brain blasts at me. I'm prepared to shove people out of my way, but they are actually parting like that sea in the Bible. I slump down and take Caroline's head from the hands of a faceless dad. Blood covers her bluish face and trails across the pavement. A siren blares.

"Holly! Wilson! Go get our bag! Bring it to me. Run! It has the Ativan shot in it."

A crowd is hovering around us, peering down at a convulsing, bleeding Caroline. Billy and I hold onto her, trying to prevent more physical trauma and humiliation. The Ativan shot is not really a shot; it's an anal plunger. It's the fastest and safest way for us to get the drugs into her system and stop the seizure.

Thinking I am going to need to administer this drug in front of this swarm of people, I try to keep Caroline's head on my lap while rolling her onto one side. Wilson appears with the shot in his hand, staring down at his little sister. Thankfully, just before I have to bare my daughter to the sheltering globe of eyeballs, the seizure ceases and her body goes limp. She gasps for air and proceeds to widely open and close her jaw. Her teeth clang together as she tries to gulp down oxygen.

"Oh Holly," I cry out. "Her favorite earrings. One is gone."

I think back to Christmas, only eight months ago. I had splurged on those earrings because I knew they were perfect for her. Elegant white gold, twisted loops; I was right, she wore them every day. I frantically begin searching for the earring. It seems to be the most important task at the moment. I cannot let her lose one more thing. When the ambulance arrives and they load her onto the stretcher, I walk beside her with the paramedics.

Holly calls out, "Don't worry, Mom, I'll keep looking. We will find the earring."

Caroline still has a scar from that day. And only one white gold, twisted loop earring.

CHAPTER 8
A CHEETAH DRESSED IN ANN TAYLOR

It's Monday morning and I have unraveled from the pool trauma into an insecure, fruitless place. Fixated on what the other swim team moms must think, I'm convinced they are wondering how a mother could have her epileptic daughter out there on the hot pavement. They think if they were me, their daughter would have been at home, or in a wheelchair, wearing a helmet.

And to top it off, where was Caroline's mother when she fell? Why, lounging on a chair on the other side of the pool, that's where. I don't want to care what the hell they think, but as hard as I am fighting for my daughter, for my family, I fear they are right. I should never have sat down and taken my eye off the ball, even for one minute.

These insecurities needle at me, suggesting I don't deserve even a tiny taste of joy until I win the war on seizures and put my family back together like a Hallmark movie. These self-imposed restrictions are affecting all aspects of my life. Workdays are no longer energizing. My work—engaging in competition, building bonds with customers, giving inspiring speeches from a stage—was once a joyful energy that is now a pernicious memory. Each day I put on the clothes that used to make me feel feminine and strong: a bright-colored suit with a unique flair, chunky heels, and funky earrings. But now, the same clothes feel like a costume. I wear it as armor hoping it will carry the old Tara into work, leaving my pain and fear in the Explorer.

The people in the high schools I service are not just customers, they are friends. And so, as soon as I enter a school's front office, the friends want to sit and talk or pray with me. Through pleading eyes, they ask, "How is Caroline?" Then, "How are you?" And often, it is followed with the dreaded *clutch-and-tilt*. They gently clutch my arm, tilt their head, and say, "Really, how *are* you?"

The entire time, I'm keeping one eye on my phone. I just want to do the job I came to do and race back home to Caroline as fast as I can. But so many loving, concerned friends want to express their sorrow and support. I want to show gratitude and be present with them, but the fear of a call from Oconee County Middle School keeps me tense with my heartrate clanging in overdrive. I fake my wide smile, agreeing that God is in charge and, "Yes, of course, everything happens for a reason."

But inside my head I yell, *Fuck that. I'm in charge now. I will never accept this.*

When the war is won, and my family is church-portrait perfect, I will sit down, breathe again, and recall joy back into my life.

It's September 19, 2005. I'm driving home from a long day of sales presentations, heartfelt prayers, relentless tension, and many clutch-and-tilts. As I drive out of Lincoln County, my flip phone gets a signal and the voicemails load. I see the one I am waiting for—Dr. Fripp's office. Earlier this morning, I had finally given in to desperation and called his office. As much as I blame him for blowing up Caroline's life, I set my rage aside to ask for help.

Research has become my obsession. My relentless focus on finding answers, doctors, therapies, and procedures has me locked out of living and chained me to the goal of a seizure-free Caroline. Maybe Dr. Fripp could get us off this drug trial train we are on at Emory University. I return the call to his office as I make my way through Oglethorpe County. His receptionist stammers when she hears my voice, "Yes, yes. Dr. Fripp will call you as soon as he finishes with his patients. Mrs. Heaton, he was so glad to get your message. He will call you back shortly. We are all praying for Caroline."

Just as I pull into the driveway, Dr. Fripp's office number pops up on my phone. I leave everything in the Explorer and sit down on our screened porch to take the call. A locomotive turns up my heartrate. Sitting on the porch swing, my foot shoves the swing as high as the space will allow.

Curtly, I explain to Dr. Fripp why I've contacted him. "I need to stop Caroline's seizures. Her life is crumbling before my eyes. The people at Emory just keep drugging her. I need options and I don't know where to begin."

I can't stop what comes ripping off my tongue next. "Dr. Fripp," my voice cracks and the swing bangs into the porch beams behind me. "I want to know. I believe that if you had come to the office that day when Sherri asked you to, we would not be having this conversation. She said she thought the rash looked unusual. I think if you had come to the office that day, you would have prescribed steroids and Caroline would be perfectly fine today. But you didn't; you didn't come."

With a shaky inhale, I grip the swing's chain and bite into my bottom lip. Through the phone I hear the kind, gentle voice of the most beloved pediatrician in the community.

Patiently, compassionately, Dr. Fripp assures me of three things. Administering steroids is an aggressive option and had he come, he still would not have suggested it. Perhaps some doctors would have, but that would not have been his recommendation. And then, he offers a genuine, intentional apology. He clearly, sincerely regrets not coming that day, not because he would have done anything differently, but because of the hurt it has caused. He then makes a promise, "What we need to do now is help Caroline. I have a lot of people I want to reach out to. I will do that tonight. If you let me, I will take the lead on looking for answers, options from the top experts in the field of epilepsy. I will call you back first thing tomorrow morning with some recommendations of where to go and who to see."

The call ends and hope flickers. Kathleen comes to mind, because she worked for Dr. Fripp for many years. She is a discriminating woman who is loyal to those she respects. Kathleen thinks the world of Dr. Fripp and trusts him without question.

As I close the phone, I sense something slipping away. It's a force that I have been using to charge at life like a starving cheetah. It's anger, the kind of anger that is fueled by condemnation. It's uncomfortable to imagine letting go of this energy of rage, yet in this moment, I see what I have been missing. I miss myself. The reflection in my mirror has become a somber-faced woman with a forced smile who feeds on a fury born of blame.

The porch swing has stopped. My naked feet are resting on top of my black pumps. Tears trickle down my cheeks. "Thank you, Dr. Fripp," I whisper. It's time to return to the Tara who doesn't rely on the toxic energy of blame to keep her fighting spirit alive.

Accusation is a form of self-victimization, when you think about it. It was tarring my soul. It is safer to blame Dr. Fripp for Caroline's state, because it lets me off the hook. But in exchange, I abandoned the promise I had made to myself long ago: *I will give no one the power to break my spirit.* I realize in this moment that I had almost relinquished that power to Dr. Fripp. His sorrow is deep and real; and now he is going to help my little girl. A surge of hope shoots me off the porch swing and into the house. Let's see if we can do a little dancing while I prepare my famous pizza salad for dinner.

The next morning, I stay at home to await Dr. Fripp's call, because I want to focus and I need a strong cell signal. I sit on the porch ready and waiting—coffee, cigarettes, phone, notepad, and pen. This phone call will set me on a new path toward beating seizures. It's the call that will keep hope alive.

I wait. And I wait. More coffee. Another cigarette. And another. I check the phone. Again. And again. In complete disbelief, I conclude he's not going to call. He's not showing up for Caroline. Again. At around 10:30, I call his office. The line is busy. Well, that is odd. I have never heard that. I guess something is wrong with the phone. And then, Kathleen calls.

"Hey," I snap. I hear nothing. "Kathleen? Hello?" Kathleen breaks the latch on her throat. "Dr. Fripp! He, he . . . . . . " She sobs out a few more words, "He was out running early this morning. He was hit by a car. He was killed."

CHAPTER 9
THE MAGNET SCRAMBLE

A few months after Dr. Fripp's tragic death, I looked into the eyes of Caroline's neurologist at the Emory Clinic and verbalized my frustration for the last time.

"Dr. Fleischer, look at Caroline. She's right here, and she's not. This is not our Caroline. She's lethargic, dazed, and confused. And the drugs aren't working! Could we possibly get her off these drugs and try to manage the seizures? Maybe they could go away if we didn't keep drugging her, causing her to need them more."

Dr. Fleischer's response fuels me to this very day, "No. Taking her off medication would be very damaging." She explained that Caroline's seizures travel across her hippocampus. With every seizure, there is damage to that region. The hippocampus is responsible for learning, for memory, and for the management of emotions. She says, "We have to find a way to stop her seizures, or they will continue to cause damage to her brain." I want to say, *Well then just get the hell out of my way, lady. I will find a way to stop these seizures.* But instead, I say, "The drugs are failing. What else is there?"

Dr. Fleischer sends us to a pediatric epileptologist, Dr. Park, in Augusta, Georgia. He wants to gather his own data and study Caroline's seizures, so we make the two-hour drive and check in for a repeat performance from Wire Woman. Caroline is admitted to the hospital where she is hooked up to the EEG machine, video cameras turned on, and her medication is drastically reduced.

When Caroline's medication is suddenly and significantly altered, only one type of seizure is expected: Tonic-Clonic (a.k.a. Grand Mal). The entire body jerks with a superhuman strength that is beyond voluntary simulation. According to Johns Hopkins Medicine, tonic activity is strong spasms of the muscles that force air out of the lungs and clonic activity is intense, rapid jerking movements that affect the face, arms, and legs.

After about 48 hours, with no warning, Caroline's entire body stiffens with a strength that could literally knock you to the ground. We try to hold her, protect her in some way. Her body convulses uncontrollably as her eyes dart back and forth with their own tiny, speedy spasms. Her torso clamps forward, her jaw is clinched, her legs are stiff and flailing wildly from her hip sockets. One arm is bent, jerking so hard that it rips at her shoulder's rotator cuff without mercy.

We press a little red button to alert the nurses. Pink scrubs with perky ponytails and button-adorned Crocs come running into the room. They remind us not to block the video camera as we all watch Caroline's face turn grayish-blue due to lack of oxygen. After about two minutes and 15 seconds, the horror subsides.

The nurses put oxygen on Caroline and tell her it's okay. I think, *Wow, this is anything but okay.* But what do I expect them to say? *Sorry, honey. Your life really does suck ass.* No, I just sit and watch Caroline recover. My esophagus constricts and swells. I'm desperate for the cheery pink scrubs to disappear so I can cradle and kiss my daughter.

We spend four and a half days on this seizure train, littered with reruns of *That's So Raven* and *Fresh Prince of Bel Air*, to-go bags of Firehouse Subs, and sneaking out for smoke breaks (okay, that's just me). The nurse tells us that, after the doctor stops by to report his findings, we will be free to leave. Like half-numb soldiers, we haphazardly pack in preparation to go home.

When the doctor arrives, we stop and sit at the edges of our seats. He tells us the studies show that Caroline is not a candidate for brain surgery, because her seizures' origins are multi-focal. At this time, focal resection surgery, which is literally removing the seizure focus from the brain, is the most common and successful type of surgery for epilepsy. The doctor says that Caroline's seizures originate from many random areas of the brain, and from both sides. So, no, surgery is not an option.

However, he recommends that she have a Vagus nerve stimulator (VNS) implanted in her chest. The Vagus nerve is the conduit that transports information from the neck, chest, and stomach to the brain and back again. Research concludes that when the Vagus nerve is electrically stimulated, it can reduce the intensity and the frequency of seizures. With a VNS implant, some patients see up to a 50 percent reduction, some are able to significantly reduce their medication, and for some, it doesn't help at all. We agree it makes sense to move forward with this low-risk procedure.

@

After the surgery, we are given a little magnet. The VNS will intermittently and automatically transmit electrical currents. When Caroline feels the premonition of a seizure, called an aura, she is supposed to run the magnet over the generator in her chest to set off a manual current. If she doesn't have an aura, or it's too brief, her nearest companion should be trained to run the magnet over the device during the seizure, because it can minimize the time span or intensity of the episode.

We keep making trips to Augusta to have the generator turned to a higher frequency and electrical current potency, because it isn't yet working. For months, with every aura, moan, or seizure, like trained lab rats, we all scramble for that magnet. But unlike lab rats, we never get a reward. Her seizures are no less frequent and no less violent. Eventually, the doctor concedes, "Vagus nerve stimulation is not going to help Caroline."

Even though I innately knew this was what we would learn, hearing it confirmed by Dr. Park feels like a zap to my last sparks of optimism. I wonder if this is how cynics are born. It is much safer to believe you won't succeed, to have low expectations and accept your circumstances.

Cynics, I imagine, develop their negativity bias to avoid being slapped across the face with defeat.

But I'm not a cynic. In fact, I've been called a Polly Anna all my life.

About a year and a half into the failure-fest that kicked off my sales career, I was crying through the phone to a Georgia colleague. He gave me some advice that day: "TH, you need to stabilize. Don't let yourself get too high when you win, and don't let yourself get too low when you lose." I respected this guy; he was one of the greatest success stories in the business, so I took his advice to heart.

After a few weeks, though, I abandoned this bullshit mentality. Some of us are not wired that way. I invest with my heart, body, and soul. It's who I am. I know I can handle defeat. I may bend into the hurt, but I won't break. So, when I hurt, it's a mental, emotional, and physical thrashing. But when there is a victory, look out, baby, because the celebration is about to unleash.

What I know is that hope is energy. Without hope, I would have fallen prey to depression, self-loathing, and feelings of immense failure. While I have always promised myself I will never give a person the power to break my spirit, I am learning that one of those people could be me. *Especially me.* If I don't keep searching and taking action, then I risk more than the temporary branding of defeat. If I stop seeking, then I let hope die, and I will have killed my spirit with my own idle hands. And so, after letting the pain of the VNS failure move through me, a fierce, more determined warrior charges on.

CHAPTER 10
FRIED PORK RINDS

My research obsession has reached a new height. I sit in the driver's seat while my sales associate, Brad, drives us to customers and prospects. Rather than taking care of my business, I make countless phone calls to level-four (top-tier) epilepsy centers, therapists, natural healing practitioners, functional medicine experts, acupuncturists, chiropractors, hydraulic chamber facilities, massage therapists, biofeedback experts, and, and, and. Nothing is off the table. No option is too far, too expensive, or too extreme to consider.

As I said, I search and I act. Billy and I decide that the next attempt will be the Ketogenic Diet. The doctor who is leading a big trial is at Johns Hopkins in Baltimore. So, yep, to Baltimore! On the path to finding a cure for refractory seizures, I'm all fight and strength. Yet . . . I'm worried that the cabin pressure of an airplane could cause seizures, so I decide to drive. I tell Caroline, "It will be fun! Two ladies on a road trip!"

But that's not my truth. My Explorer will trap me beside my daughter. I feel dread, which feels shameful.

This is an opportunity for me to act as Caroline's grief counselor and motivational coach. I know how it will go. She will pepper me with questions. Her struggle to comprehend my answers will sting me with evidence of her trickling decline. With each story from school that I can't bear to hear, I will feel her confidence leak out and slip away. But to sit in Caroline's world, to help her try to understand complex thoughts and to hear her panic with an inarticulable knowing that her friends are ostracizing her, takes a kind of strength I am not sure I'm built for.

With great detail, Caroline rehashes the stories of Katelyn telling her that no one likes her anymore, Shelby telling her she's going to be in special ed, Tricia telling her she has gotten fat, and Merri telling her that everyone says she is gross. She whimpers and she wails. She asks over and over, "Why? Why me? Why?"

Even knowing she needs to tell it, to yell it, I can't keep hearing it. I offer the only thing I know how to give—the spirit of a fighter. "I will find answers, Honey. Your life will get better. And screw those mean girls. Please just hang tough and believe me, we will stop these seizures." I take a giant breath in and with force and fire say, "I promise."

We are about seven hours into the trip when my phone rings. I recognize the area code as Washington County and suspect it might be my very best account calling. I answer it and hear, "Ms. Heaton, this is Hal Brown, the new principal at Washington County High School."

"Oh yes, Mr. Brown! Of course," I say in my best fake-cheery voice. "Congratulations on the new role! I'm not in front of my calendar right now, but as soon as I am, we can set a time to meet and go over the plans for next year."

"Actually," says Hal Brown, "I would like to set a time for you to come in and provide a presentation before we can commit to working with you in the coming school year."

My skin goes hot and my breath quickens. Not only is this high school my best revenue generating account, it is special to me. It was my first big win, when I finally started to break free and build a real business. But more precious than the win and the revenue is the extraordinary spirit of the small town of Sandersville, Georgia. I love the teachers, staff, and students; and I love how such a racially diverse rural town pulses with grateful, unassuming, celebratory students.

With a slightly shaky voice, I pretend not to know that my competitor has gotten to Hal Brown. Usually, that doesn't worry me much. I've never lost an account that I had to defend to keep. In this case however, I know I have reason to worry. Since the day Caroline went back to school, I've been racing home after every service visit. I haven't been staying and taking care of the relationships that I have built. I didn't even take the time to go and meet the brand-new principal at Washington County.

We finish the call with compulsory niceties, and I click the phone off. With the gnawing realization that I'm going to pay for neglecting this precious client, I keep driving toward a seizure-free life for Caroline.

◉

Johns Hopkins is the most impressive hospital I have ever visited (and I have been in many). Like a treasured customer, they greet you upon arrival. They provide clear, simple instructions, offer water, and express gratitude. They don't rush you; they escort you to each office or waiting room where you wait only if you are early.

We meet with the Ketogenic doctor and members of his team. After in-depth conversation and extensive review of Caroline's history, they provide all the information we need to get her into ketosis. We are to check her urine twice a day. If she doesn't eat enough fat and if she consumes any carbs outside of a little bit of broccoli or green beans, she will fall out of ketosis and this can cause immediate seizures. He shared the success of his trials—over an 80 percent chance of reducing seizures and better than a 50 percent chance of Caroline becoming seizure-free and reducing or *even eliminating* the diabolic epilepsy drugs.

Like dynamite, hope rockets through me.

Optimism spills from my mouth during the drive back home. I want Caroline to absorb it and conjure motivation so she can endure the restrictive diet. The task is massive. (This was long before Keto was a fad, so finding carb-free versions of anything outside of meat and fat was a colossal undertaking.) But I'm committed, and I believe in Caroline's fortitude. She desperately wants her life back, so she returns my high five and sentiment, "We got this, Mom."

The first step is shopping. Billy stays home with the kids, ready to pitch in when I return. Kathleen jumps in my passenger seat and I start spewing as I drive:

"Holy fuck-a-moly, Kath. This is a life-altering commitment. Everything, and I mean everything, has carbs or sugar. I will have to read every single label and refer to this big-ass Keto bible, every day for the rest of my life. And then, oh my God, look at these jacked-up recipes! If she wants chicken fingers, get this. I will coat them in *mayonnaise*, roll them in *pork rinds* and *deep fry* them. What the literal fuck? Who would eat that? I feel like I'm going to kill her trying to get her life back!"

"Duke's or Hellman's?" Kathleen asks.

"What?" I snap.

"The mayonnaise. Duke's or Hellman's? What kind do we need for the chicken fingers? I mean, not to be a snob about it, but I'm gonna need Hellman's."

I've heard Jesus can turn water into wine. Well, Kathleen can turn tears into laughter. I crack a smile, breathe in deeply, let out a chuckle, and keep talking. With a slower pace and a more rational tone, I continue, "I have lists and instructions and recipes that call for so many ingredients that I have never used. And everything must be cross-referenced in this Keto guide book. Plus, dammit, Caroline has already lost enough. I can't just feed her sausage and lettuce. I want her to enjoy her food like everyone else."

Kathleen sorts through my lists and recipes as I drive. She finally folds them up and says, "Where's the beer? It's not on the list. We're gonna need a lot of beer."

"Whatever you need, woman," I assure her. "As long as you don't abandon me, I will keep you Terrapin-ready."

"I'm here for you," she affirms. "I'm not passing up a front-row seat at your kitchen counter to watch *Cooking Gone Bad with Tara Heaton*."

We arrive at Earth Fare, the natural foods grocery store in downtown Athens. With the lists, notes, and Keto book, we slowly walk each aisle. Me with my granny glasses, I'm reading, checking, huffing, and puffing—with Kathleen in lockstep, making wisecracks about my recipes and bitching that they don't sell Hellman's.

Every time I see one of the mellow, hipster associates, I ask for help. With zero eye contact and a deadpan tone, they tell me where to find coconut flour or egg white powder. I wonder if they would be any more welcoming if they knew that I secretly envied them. I, too, want to sport a pink rooster-tail hair style, fishnet stockings, and green Doc Martins. We forge on, my hands gripping the cart like I'm driving it around a racetrack. Kathleen sees my tension, tears threatening to escape, and she whispers, "Keep your shit together. We are almost done. I saw some Marlboro Lights in your car. You can smoke one and I'll hang my head out the window the whole way home."

By the time we approach the check-out line, I'm biting my lip to keep it from quivering. My mind is spewing with doubt. What have I done? I'm already working beyond my capacity, trying to take care of three kids, their needs, their problems, their activities, their social lives, their doctors' appointments, their meltdowns—all while running a highly competitive business. Have I lost my mind? How will I find time to devote to this?

We start piling all the groceries onto the tiny conveyor belt. I see dreadlocks spill down on top of a tattoo-covered arm. I look up at the face that belongs to these artistic extremities, but I get distracted trying to imagine if I could fit my whole bologna log right through her stretched-out earlobe. She reminds me of a dream catcher. Before she will scan the first item, she raises her pierced eyebrow and asks, "Did you bring your own bags? We don't do bags. You know, for Mother Earth."

And just like that, I crack. I start crying right there, as the edgy dream catcher looks at me as if I'm officially her worst suburban, soccer-mom nightmare.

Back home, with Kathleen by my side (okay, well, sitting at my kitchen counter, coaching, counseling, and cackling), Billy and I are able to make this Keto diet a way of life for Caroline. And what a champion she is. She will not be tempted to deviate from the menu. If anyone offers her as much as a mini-Reese's cup (her favorite), she declines. She eats fatty meats, more meats, fried anything and everything. I keep a log of every morsel she consumes, count every fat gram, and every tiny carb. The proof is the visible weight loss and in her urine. Twice a day, she pees on a little piece of litmus paper called a ketone strip, to assure us that she is maintaining ketosis.

For four months, we continue this diet with one hundred percent devotion. It's time for a final check-in with Johns Hopkins. I'm hoping that a doctor from such a magical facility is going to have something more, a secret hack saved only for the rare people who have refractory seizures. But no, he only expresses his sympathy for the unsuccessful attempt. He explains:

"Some people just don't respond to ketosis. You've done a perfect job. Caroline is just one of those rare cases. You can return to her normal diet immediately."

CHAPTER 11
STONE-COLD CHEER MOM

Before encephalitis, I had the mental and physical strength to keep my business running and still show up as the mom with snack bags, checks, permissions slips, doctor notes, and science projects. I raced to recitals, ballgames, competitions, awards programs, teacher conferences, and on and on and on.

The load of responsibilities was already showing its effects. Holly had anxiety before it was the universal epidemic it is today. Wilson's competitive, intense nature had turned away from academics and toward sports and socializing. Ironically, I was least worried about Caroline. She wasn't as anxious and intense as Holly and Wilson. She had a lot of friends, made good grades, and was active. My only worry about her, even more ironically, was that she was growing up too fast, too interested in boys at such a young age, and as my mom would call it, "running with the fast crowd."

Our turbo-charged schedule created a pandemonium that I welcomed. Without hesitation, I soaked up life as an energetic, passionate working mom of three kids. I took pride in giving every ounce of myself to each day. *It was a joy that felt earned.*

Now Billy has added tutor and education advocate to his plate and I have added neurology ninja to mine. With this added weight of fighting to rehabilitate Caroline's life, Wilson and Holly are being neglected. It's not intentional, but I am undeniably aware of it. Holly takes second place to my desperate obsession to stop Caroline's seizures, partly because she is the baby and partly because she is vocal about her needs. But she still gets only a fraction of the mom I used to be. Even when I'm with her, my mind is drilling down on stopping her sister's decline. Wilson, on the other hand, is not expressing any need. He insists he is fine and available to help carry the weight of Caroline's impaired cognition, dangers to her safety, and torment of her daily life.

Like a clearly defined archetype, I can see the mom that Wilson and Holly need. But I can't give her to them. It would be easy to blame lack of time or fatigue, but those feel like cheap excuses. The taste of the truth is sour, rotten from my inside. I'm too weak. So I barricade myself from my own children. The thought of cradling them and absorbing their pain petrifies me, because I'm afraid it will break me.

Caroline is starting her ninth-grade year, so she has joined her now eleventh-grade brother at the high school.

Billy, Wilson, and I are sitting in the high school assistant principal's office. Mr. Powell says, "Wilson. We have a zero-tolerance policy for fighting. I should expel you. That means you go to alternative school, and you give up football, soccer, and FFA. But considering what your family is going through, I'm going to make an exception. You will be allowed to go to In-School Suspension one more time. This is your final chance."

With a solemn face, I stare at this clean-shaven, plumpish man who has shiny, black hair. His matching mustache dances to the rhythm of his southern drawl. He holds up a carbon-copied piece of paper and continues, "The pink slip says Trace McNeal touched your Pop-Tart? That's why you, it says, *slammed him into the wall and threatened his safety* in the football locker room?"

I look over at Wilson. With elbows on his knees and his forearm muscles and veins bulging, he stares at his feet.

"He deserved it," Wilson mutters.

Mr. Powell's calm drawl continues like an HR mouthpiece, "Now, Wilson. I don't know what really went on there, but surely you didn't assault Trace because," and he air quotes with his giant hands, "he touched your Pop-Tart."

"He hurt my sister!" Wilson explodes as he unclasps his hands and wipes tears and snot from his face. "He and his friends. They keep making fun of her. I have to protect her. She's my sister!" He puts his head back down and Billy grips his shaking shoulders.

"Now, son," Powell starts. "Your job here at Oconee County High School is to focus on your studies and your extra-curricular activities. Leave the discipline to us. We don't tolerate bullyin' of any sort."

I look up in agreement as if I'm Team Powell. But I think, *What a load of shit. This is supposed to be one of the best high schools in the state of Georgia. Yet everyday now, Caroline comes home and collapses in tears.*

I try to keep listening to this lecture but my mind drifts to Caroline before epilepsy. Her fifth- and sixth-grade teachers each told us she has a real heart for the underdog. On countless occasions, Caroline had left her group of friends on the playground or in the cafeteria to join a student who was alone. And her seventh-grade teacher even called Billy, all teary to say:

"You have one extraordinary child, Mr. Heaton. Caroline is in this so-called popular crowd. Today I watched her walk away from their table, *with her lunch*, and go sit down beside Anne Rowell. Poor Anne, she is always alone. Until today."

These old memories are in dark contrast to what happened just yesterday. At lunch time, Caroline went to sit at the crowded table of ninth graders she innocently still believed were her friends. The biggest one, Kyle, stood up as she approached. She set her lunch down, and just as she attempted to relax into the blue plastic chair, Kyle snatched it out from under her. As planned, she tumbled to the ground, the weight of her backpack helping to bruise her tailbone.

Back to the current moment in this meeting with Wilson, Billy, and the principal, my thoughts spiral: *Do your fucking job, man. Put a stop to this bullying and protect Wilson's sister. Then maybe he can take your idealistic advice and focus on his future.*

After the two-mile drive home, I put the Explorer into park, look over at my son and beg him to come back to me. "Wilson, what is wrong? You are so angry. You lack motivation. That has never been you."

Wilson shrugs.

That's it. That's all I get. With a fanatical desperation, I press on, "Please talk to me. Or talk to someone. Let me take you to a counselor."

He puts his hand on the door handle and says, "I'm fine, Mom."

Wilson is opening the door and fumbling for his keys. He opens his own little truck door where I get a glimpse of fast-food garbage, energy drink cans, and tobacco tins strewn about. He looks up at me, but doesn't meet my eyes as he says, "Mom, I promise I'm fine. I'm good. I'm going to the ag barn to feed my pig and then I'm going to ride horses and spend the night with Ethan. I will see you later. I love you." And with that, his engine roars and he screeches out of the driveway at the speed of anger.

I too, want to speed away. Wilson is running, not coping, not dealing. They say kids learn more from watching their parents than from any crap that comes out of our mouths.

A very old memory appears in my mind. It was the day my dad moved out, making my parents' divorce official. I was 11. It was one of two times in my life I saw my father with tears in his eyes. While I sat in the kitchen, my mom walked him out to his car. When she returned, her eyes were red-rimmed and glossy. She reached for her cigarettes, and before disappearing into her office, she told me what had just happened in the driveway. Before my dad got behind the wheel, he had made a fist and punched the side of his car, again and again, repeating the words, "I hate my father. I hate him." My father had inherited his father's traits, traits that were costing him his family.

Wilson is inheriting my traits and I wonder what it will cost him. Here I sit, begging my son to stop telling himself he is fine and to accept some help. But I'm not in therapy, I don't slow down, and we all know I'm not fine, either. I'm running at top speed, fighting the war on epilepsy. But I'm not just running toward a cure; I'm running away, away from heartache. I try to fight it off with constant movement, commitments, activities—and when there's nowhere left to run, I smoke it away in any hiding place I can find.

My Explorer is the best hiding place. I fire up a cigarette and ruminate on how to do better for Wilson. But how? Won't forcing him to stay home and witness more seizures and despair only intensify his grief? I realize I don't have an answer. I guess this is what counselors are for, so I decide to find one for Wilson.

I try to smoke away the anguish while driving across town to pick up Holly from cheerleading. I think about how many times I have made this drive.

Recalling one weekend in particular makes me wonder how in the hell I became a cheer mom. I was sitting on the floor of a massive convention center with all the other mothers. The cheerleaders were prancing around, all hopped up on sugar from eating their goody-bags full of candy for lunch and Dippin' Dots for dessert. Every time I found myself spending my weekend in some expensive hotel, covered in glitter, dragging around a toolbox full of makeup and hair paraphernalia, I questioned my judgment.

And so, on this day, I asked the other mom-servants, "Look at us, y'all. We drive back and forth to the gym every day all week and then we spend our entire weekend here to basically serve our daughters, all for a two-minute-and-thirty-second performance. Do you ever ask yourselves, 'Why are we doing this?'"

And at that moment I got the answer I will never forget. The mom of the tiniest princess with the longest blonde hair stared at me with shock and asked, "Tara. Don't you want your girls to be cheerleaders in high school?"

My mouth opened to reply, but I didn't say aloud the response in my head: *Fuck no, I do not!*

I'm still fearing this fate as I pull into the cheer gym parking lot. Holly was seven years old when she declared that she wanted to take a tumbling class. I found a class at this gym, but I made it clear to Holly, "No cheerleading. You can take tumbling classes. That's it." She was delighted, so we signed her up. God, was I naïve.

I spray myself with Moonlit Path from Bath and Body Works, swish some Scope, look around for other mom-servants, discreetly spit the mouthwash into the gravel, and walk in to watch my baby girl. The gym is bustling with tumbling passes, workouts, and dance routines, but I don't see Holly or her squad. The receptionist sees my confusion and says, "They didn't hit their pyramid, so they had to go outside and run two miles."

I sit down in a little metal chair and wait, wondering how running in the heat will help these children improve their pyramid prowess.

As the girls come panting and moaning back into the gym, I expect to see the Holly who has become a powerful tumbling athlete. And then I see her, a bit behind the rest of the pack. But she's not the Holly I know. The big, round, brown eyes that used to dance brightly are weary. The arms that used to give hugs with all their might dangle beneath tense shoulders that used to stand fearlessly straight and welcome the world with wonder.

Even though she is only feet away from me, looking at her makes me long for her. Part of me wants to run to her, as if I can revive the dreaming bundle of light she used to be. My heart wants to hold her, breathe her in, and tell her it will all be okay. But I'm afraid to free this part of me.

As we drive home from the gym, Holly reminds me that we leave in three weeks to drive to Florida for a cheer competition. "Mom, please can you ask Dad to stay home with Caroline? When she is there, you are never really with me and the other moms. Plus, it's awkward how she tries to be friends with my friends. Mom, please."

Holly continues to make her case as we walk into the house. I interrupt her to tell Michelle, Caroline's caregiver, goodbye. Michelle informs me, "She had another seizure after her tutor left. She didn't fall. I was right there and I caught her. And now she is back asleep on the couch."

I hold my breath, desperate to run into the living room and get Caroline off the couch. When the brain works to shift from beta waves into the theta and delta waves of sleep, it often causes seizures. Caroline shouldn't be sleeping on a couch. If she twists one way, she could suffocate in the cushions, and if she twists the other way, she will fall.

Not taking the time to explain this to Michelle, I rush her out the door and turn to get quickly to Caroline's side. Holly keeps pressuring me about leaving her sister at home for the next cheer competition. As I dart past her on the way to the living room, Holly yells, "Mom! I'm talking to you. I was talking to you. This was important to me! But you never listen. You are only worried about Caroline. Michelle said she was fine!"

Before I can apologize—a daily ritual—she runs upstairs. Footsteps thunder down the hall. A door slams. A second door slams. Then stomping back across the hall and from the top of the stairs, Holly yells, "Where is Wilson? Why is he never here? You just let him go wherever he wants! I hate it here too, you know."

I want to yell back up at Holly that I am doing my very best and that some kids have it worse. Why do we remind our children that kids are starving in Africa when they express their needs? Holly is starving for comfort, but I can't force my legs to run up the stairs to hold her and allow her tears to soak into me. I swallow the hurt and focus on what must be done in the moment. I try to move Caroline slowly onto the floor without waking her. Damn, no luck. She wakes up. I tell her to just rest so I can start dinner. But no, she needs to unload the pain of her day, too.

As I boil pasta and chop broccoli, she sits at the kitchen table, spewing a rapid-fire litany of disappointments. "I asked Brianna to spend the night this weekend, but she said she is going to her grandmother's. But I know she lied, because Chloe told me she is going to the movies with her. So I asked Clara to find out why they didn't invite me. I said I bet it's because of my seizures. But Clara said no, they said it's because I'm dumb now."

My brain and heart are at war; logic tells me she needs to let this out, while my heart wants to beg her to stop. I look up from the broccoli and fight my urge to disappear. Instead, I block the impending cry of "Why me?"

Dropping the knife on the cutting board, I dart past the counter to Caroline's side. Determination sears through my pores. "Caroline," I say. "Hang tough, my angel. I've found another doctor. She is amazing. I think she is going to help you. Just believe me. We won't stop until you get your life back."

Caroline looks up at me as her face softens, her eyes grow wide, her lips separate. It's as if I have tossed her a life preserver, a tangible symbol of hope. Seeing her suffering ease in this moment teases me with the taste of a small win.

"We are going to Los Angeles," I tell her. "We will stay there for three or four weeks and you will do something called biofeedback. This lady is one of the few people in the country who does this. We are all going out there during spring break. But you and I will stay for three or four weeks, for as long as it takes."

Billy walks in the door as I toss the meal together. I give him the rundown, all facts, no emotion. "Dinner is ready. Please leave a plate for me in the microwave. Holly is upstairs and Wilson is at Ethan's for the night. I'm going to the office to work. If Holly asks about the snacks for her National Honor Society meeting, just tell her I will get the stuff tonight at the grocery store and get up before school to make them."

I attempt to kiss Billy on the cheek as I grab my keys, but I miss. Neither of us care.

CHAPTER 12
BEST FRIENDS WITHOUT BENEFITS

And, oh yeah, I have a marriage. Even in the pre-epilepsy days, it was being neglected and functioned more like two buddies trying to run a small kids' camp.

I'm lying in my bed beside Caroline, basking in the silence that lets my mind wander. The five dusty blades of the ceiling fan hang static, reminding me of the family that was once a synchronized unit. For over two years, like a China doll, Caroline has slept beside me, motionless, until I hear that familiar moan or feel her stiffen before a seizure. I imagine her lying in her own bed, seizing all alone, with no one to make sure she comes out of it, no one to comfort her, and tell her she is safe. It is simply incomprehensible. And so, she sleeps with me and Billy sleeps in her room at the opposite end of the hall.

I reach over, caress Caroline's head and think about Billy sleeping soundly in her bed. You would think we would miss sleeping together, that he would complain about not sleeping with his wife. But no. We never mention it. I finally accepted that Billy is not naturally affectionate. I used to try to snuggle up to him, to hold him, or to be held. I used to long for intimacy from him, the warmth of touch, but now I don't. Not anymore.

Do I miss affection? Romance? Sex? Oh yes, I dream of it. And when I dream of it, an inkling of shame trickles in. I'm convinced that other moms would not desire intimacy and romance if they had a child suffering like mine. Other moms would be solely, one-dimensionally the mother of a child with special needs. Would Caroline be better off with another mom? Idealizing other mothers brings a cold, gray version of myself into focus—dutiful and methodical, nurturing a declining Caroline while I accept the fate of more seizures, more drugs, on repeat.

Would I be softer, more present for Wilson and Holly if I simply followed the protocol that is allotted by our insurance and the local providers? My obsession with beating seizures is stealing their mother from their lives. I justify my actions by believing that winning the war on seizures will be a win for our whole family, not just for Caroline. I trust in what my spirit needs to keep fighting while swatting away the shame of not showing up fully for my other children. For us to be the best moms we can be, we have to understand our wiring. I know how I am wired. I'm not made for slow and steady. The way I approach life brings a greater risk of crashing down in defeat. But it's the only way I know how to keep going—by going for the gold.

My going-for-the-gold spirit lets the girl in me dream. When Caroline's life is back on track, free of seizures, I will be more present and intentional with Wilson and Holly.

But the family will change because, while I see a seizure-free life letting me fall back in love with being a mom, I don't see it catapulting me back in love with my husband. The dream is an easy divorce where Billy and I stay friends and we can each find love again. But the thought of breaking up this family, slinging more heartache at my children, is inconceivable. And so, we just keep up the façade and play our roles as directors of the three campers and their mounting needs.

But I can't convince myself I'm still in love with a man because he is kind and loyal. I hear people try to quantitatively affirm their love like a pros and cons listicle assignment. Billy is generous, thoughtful, hard-working, honest, and dependable. Should I attempt to quantify my love for Billy, there would be only one item in the con column, and it is the harsh truth. I no longer desire my husband.

I'm glad I don't have to pretend to want to kiss him goodnight. We do pretend-kiss, though, as a greeting or a bid goodbye. It's a kind of air kiss where lips miss lips and awkwardly aim toward a cheek. I liken it to greeting your grandmother at Thanksgiving while she is busy with her hands up the turkey's ass. It makes me feel sad, like I must be without sex appeal, like an Edith Bunker. But it's become part of our tag-team dance; Billy gives me the cheek and I dust against it, really only kissing myself.

I wonder, *Are we just using each other?*

We have mastered the "when you get home, I'm leaving" ritual. We have even perfected tag-teaming the bathroom. I don't want to be naked or expose my sexuality to Billy.

Now, as I stare at the fan's separate blades, I accept more harsh truth—neither does he.

And yet, we are more than co-camp directors. I cannot imagine life without him. I trust him. Respect him. *Love* him. I guess this is crazy head talk. You don't get to divorce your husband and keep him as your BFF.

A BFF connection begins with fun. When the two of you are together, fun happens. It's organic and unintentional. That was the beginning of falling in love with Billy. Even through the younger years of parenting, together we could make a trip to the Golden Pantry—the local gas station and corner store—fun. But now, I think we both deny ourselves fun. We have stored it in the attic where it waits in darkness. It's waiting for us to stamp out seizures. That single victory will free us to release fun back into our lives. I fall asleep remembering raw laughter. Denying myself fun seems my duty right now, but a revelation is seeping into my dreams.

Our kids are watching, learning. They absorb my coping skills, something I swore I would never inherit from my own mother. It wasn't that I wanted her to pretend to have fun. I wanted her to free herself to embody it. My mom was on the sidelines of her kids' fun: on the deck while we swam, on the bench while we rode rollercoasters, hunched over her sewing machine while we played card games in the den. It's why I used to ride the rides, play in the pool, make up games, and dance in the kitchen with my kids. While it may be acceptable for me to deny myself fun, I can't subscribe to the same for my kids. And yet, as I avoid their father, let the CD player grow dust, and refuse to warm a seat on our sofa, they are watching.

I consider couples therapy for a moment. But then I ask myself, *To what end?* So I can do a better job of fooling our kids? No, I don't want to fool anyone. Starting with myself and especially my children. Truth is freedom. I believe I already have the truth.

CHAPTER 13
BLACK BETTY

Even with the mastery of the tag-team duet, there are times when neither Billy nor I can be at home. Wilson is my go-to safety supervisor for Caroline. But when Wilson is unavailable, I lean on an 11-year-old girl to manage her older sister's seizures.

Holly hates to be left at home alone with Caroline. Deep down, I know that leaving her to *babysit* her big sister is probably scarring her in ways that I avoid considering. I make excuses, to myself and to her. It's in this trap that she is forced to face the slow decline of Caroline's cognitive ability. She's confined to a front-row seat to witness the life that she once coveted become one filled with doctors, tutors, and therapists—devoid of friends, mischief, creativity, or growth. The little sister is suddenly the big sister.

As Caroline's big sister role deteriorates, so does the quiet confidence she used to possess. That easy-going, yet resolute young girl still shows up every morning in the same flawless skin, dainty profile, and lips that a painter would envy. But her posture now droops, folds inward.

Her eyes idle with a grayish hue, like chocolate covered in freezer burn. She regularly begs in desperation to be around teenagers who were once her friends. They push her away, almost run from her, but she cannot accept it. It's the old analogy of putting your hand on a hot stove. She keeps going back to touch the stove and it continues to scorch her. But she remembers a once warm stove that offered inviting aromas and fulfilling experiences, so she keeps touching it, hoping it will somehow stop burning and give her back the pleasure it once produced.

We are at the middle school football game, watching Holly cheer. It's pretty hot for early April. I let Caroline come along, but I'm determined not to let her out of my sight.

Caroline begs, "Please Mom, please. Let me go over and hang out with my friends."

But I take my usual stance and just let her hate me. I know those kids will cause her to come back to me in tears. I'm also too worried about letting go of the back of her shirt. I walk across the parking lot toward the bleachers with my hand at the small of Caroline's back. I have her shirt pulled tightly and twisted into a handle for me to grip. Her frozen brown eyes smolder with contempt for me.

The band, the cheerleaders, and the coaches' whistles bombard my eardrums. The people surrounding us are smiling, hugging, laughing, and telling stories. I see all these carefree people: moms with Diet Cokes and Brighton tote bags, dads with ball caps and Blackberries, teenagers with Gatorades and Sour Punch Straws. I try to smile and wave, but it feels forced, coming from a cold place where I just try to keep my heart beating. I'm desperate to get this over with.

Keep walking, keep walking, I tell myself. No stopping to invite conversation, interrogation. We approach the bleachers and I look up. They are hard silver slats, glistening in the hot sun. Caroline starts to climb, but my grip tightens, restraining her with her little Abercrombie polo shirt.

"Let's sit down here, on the bottom bench, where we are closest to Holly," I say to Caroline in my fake-cheery voice. "We can see her better down here."

"I'm not stupid, Mom," she snaps, as she plops down beside me in a huff.

And there we sit. Me, forcing a smile directly at Holly, cheering when she holds up the smallest, blondest, tannest girls from the bottom of the pyramid and when she throws her powerful tumbling passes. But I never clap. I can't let go of Caroline's shirt. So many of the free people stop by to say hello, each giving me the clutch-and-tilt.

"Really, how *are* you," they ask as their eyes avoid mine. And then always, "I'm praying for your family. Caroline is still on our prayer list at church."

Most people move along quickly. Perhaps it's an unconscious effort to avoid getting too close to a reality they cannot imagine. If I were them, and one of them me, I'm sure I wouldn't know what to say, or how to be supportive. *Then again, maybe I am creating these awkward exchanges.*

Maybe they move along quickly because they sense I
am simply a shell of the person I used to be. I used to go
out into the world with an intentional effort of spreading
joy. I inherited this gift from my mom, the most sincere,
loving person I've ever known. While she could rarely
receive or embrace joy, giving it to others defined her.
She could find unique gifts and beauty in every person
she met, and she would shower them with compliments
about anything from the shape of their lips to the
enthusiasm in their voice. If she knew you, she would
compliment your integrity, talents, or brilliance. I used to
be just like that. But now, I'm a stiff, tense woman trying
to make it to the end of the day, alone on my back porch
with my Marlboro Light.

It's close to halftime when Katey sees us and walks
over. I love Katey. We are nothing alike, but I respect how
much she gives of herself to her family and others. Her
daughters are both cheerleaders, and her oldest, Kally, is
a longtime friend of Wilson. Unlike the other moms, after
she gives us the obligatory clutch-and-tilt, she doesn't
leave. She is genuine and compassionate, unafraid of getting close to our pain.

After a bit of small talk, she says, "Tara, I'm sorry
about Wilson. About Kally and Wilson, and the homecoming dance."

My heart sinks. I didn't know. Wilson was planning
to ask Kally to the dance; I guess she had turned him
down. There was a time when Wilson could have chosen
just about any girl in school to date. But over the past

year or so, he has changed. His choices, his appearance, his friends. I know he is getting in trouble at school, and I know he is in constant jeopardy of not passing his classes. He is also migrating toward a very different group of friends. He defends them, telling me that lower income doesn't mean lower character. I can't argue with that; I taught him that. But his friends are into partying and on the rare occasion that they do come around, they avoid me.

And now, as I sit here on this bench, the truth crystallizes in my mind. Kally doesn't want to be seen with my son, or she doesn't feel safe with him. In a way that feels sickening to admit, I don't blame her.

Katey continues to make some excuses about her daughter wanting to go to homecoming with her girlfriends, but I am lost in thought about Wilson and how he's in a constant race to avoid pain. As I'm thinking about this, no longer listening to Katey, I guess my hand loosened up on the little Abercrombie polo.

Caroline catapults into the gravel. Katey shrieks.

"No!" I drop to my knees and pull Caroline's face out of the dirt. I hold onto her as she seizes, and Katey magically pulls a T-shirt out of her tote bag. I grab it and try to stop the bleeding from Caroline's chin. People are crowded around, asking to call 911, discussing what to do to help.

The only thing I can say is, "No. No ambulance. I will be able to get her out of here, just give us about ten minutes."

As if in an action movie, I hear a familiar voice, one that makes this shit show I'm living bearable. It's Kathleen.

She pulls up to us in her Toyota minivan. She drove that big, blue grocery-getter right up to the bleachers because, well, because she is Kathleen.

She immediately takes over. "No, no ambulance. We've got her. She needs stitches. Let's get her to my van. Some of these strong young boys are looking useless." She arbitrarily selects two eighth-grade boys to help lift Caroline and they swiftly lay her in my lap in the backseat of the van.

As we start to drive away, I look up from Caroline in time to see Holly standing beside us. Kathleen rolls her window down and I say, "I'm so sorry, Holly. Please ask Julie's mom to take you home with them. I will pick you up when we get back."

"She already offered, mom," Holly says. "It's fine."

I nod and Kathleen drives us out of the parking lot. My heart pulls my eyes down to Caroline. Then back out at Holly. Then into the rearview mirror and, for a moment, I lock eyes with Kathleen.

"Bitch, we've got this," she says. As we speed toward St. Mary's, Kathleen cranks up the CD player. I hear Ram Jam boom about "Black Betty" and a child, a child that's gone wild. This tune starts to revive and comfort Caroline because the familiar sound lets her know where she is.

In a groggy slur, she says, "Miss Kathleen?"

I look again into the rearview mirror. The reflection is Kathleen in her purple sunglasses, bopping to the beat. A distant but familiar part of me faintly transforms my face. It's a smile.

CHAPTER 14
LIFE MINUTES

I found a therapist for Wilson. It took some *persuading* to get him to go; he agreed to go in exchange for the privilege of keeping his truck. But so far, it just feels like an exercise in self-congratulatory parenting. He tries to tell the therapist what she wants to hear until the time he can prove that he doesn't need counseling. During most of my childhood, my mom was in and out of therapy. She always came home with puffy eyes, a soggy tissue, and an offering of something like waffles or Frosted Flakes for dinner. I didn't get it. As I got older, I asked her why she thought it necessary to track back over trauma. She explained to me that if we don't work through our shit, one day it will sneak up and bite us in the ass.

I tell myself, *once this trauma is behind us, maybe I will model what I ask of my son and get a therapist.* As long as they don't give me the clutch-and-tilt, I may be up for it. The problem is that this war on seizures is taking longer than I anticipated. I don't think I can continue putting everything and everyone else on ice. The stifling existence is starting to stir inside me. I'm trying to figure out how to at least delight in some moments with my children. I want to stop seeing joy as a luxury I have yet to earn. So every once in a while, I let life be now.

It's a warm Saturday afternoon. The sky is clear blue, dolloped with a few white clouds. With every breeze, rusty-orange dust and the occasional dandelion puff float by. The wannabe cowboy crowd is stomping, spitting, and cupping their mouths as they holler from the metal bleachers, "Git it boy" or "Rope 'er, little mama!"

Scents of leather, tobacco, popcorn, hotdogs, and manure waft and linger. The announcer is relentless. He yells into the microphone, "She roped that little baby like she was born on a horse. That little sister is goin' places, y'all." The crowd, the announcer, the animals, and the Garth Brooks tunes all wail in tandem, producing the racket of rodeo.[1]

Wilson is devoted to bulls and broncos, declaring that he will be a bull rider for life—the life of a renegade and a nomad.

Billy, Holly, Caroline, and I remain arm-locked together on the bottom bleacher. The four of us are jacked-up on adrenaline and a heat-charged love for Wilson. Sitting on this bleacher, holding Caroline extra close, I look to my other side and drink in the old familiar smile that's dancing across Holly's face. She's not watching the rodeo, though; she's watching her brother. She can't see his face because of the helmet. With the hodgepodge of sounds, she can't hear him, either. But her eyes tell her he is alive

---

[1] A personal note: This memory took place long before I let myself see the reality of life for many rodeo animals. I am in no way an advocate for these events today.

with anticipation. He bounces, he stretches, he adjusts his chaps, snaps his glove, and taps his spurs.

On this day, I am overwhelmed with a yearning, a grieving. For Caroline? For Holly? No, for me. I miss myself. From my core, I feel my old, faithful flame. Right here in this minute, it's flickering with gratitude. I hear Garth Brooks murmur about how lightning strikes and thunder rolls as I pulse with a desire to celebrate. I think, *I'm ropin' this in. No caution, no thoughts of yesterday or tomorrow. This is joy. Dive in.*

I reach over, grab Holly's face and smooch in her whole cheek. I let go of her arm, pick up her hand, and kiss the little knuckles that she knows I adore. She rolls her eyes that are glistening in a way that I feared was only a memory. She can't conceal her smile or deny the connected happiness of right now.

As I float about in this moment, I remain rooted in reality. The reality is that we are seated in an epileptic trigger-storm. People often ask me what brings on Caroline's seizures—activity, heat, noise, stress, excitement—basically, life. Getting off the couch and living life—that's what triggers Caroline's seizures. As stress or excitement increases, the chance for a seizure heightens.

So it's no wonder Caroline has never made it through a rodeo without having a seizure. Billy and I are on guard. We keep glancing at each other, tightening the clasp of our arms linked through Caroline's. The best we can hope for is that she gets lucky and has the seizure long enough before Wilson rides, so that her postictal state will have subsided, and she can see her brother bust out of the chute and try to ride that bull. She often misses the ride completely and is then crushed. But on a few occasions, the seizure comes during the calf roping or the bronco riding and she has a chance to recover.

Today is a lucky day. We feel her body freeze and begin to stiffen. Billy and I brace ourselves and protect Caroline with our arms and shoulders as Holly puts her head down. After about 90 seconds, Caroline starts the familiar slurping and gasping for air. I check her jeans quickly. Good, they are dry. Holly pulls a hand towel from my giant purse, and I wipe the drool and sweat from her sister's face.

After about four more minutes, Caroline starts to realize where she is. She half cries, half moans in a slurred speech, "Mom! Did I miss it? Did I miss Wilson?"

Holly comforts her big sister, "No Caroline. Look. See? He's over there, still all clean and getting ready. You didn't miss it."

The announcer informs us that it's time for the finale and main event, the bull riders! Holly and I squeeze each other with excitement and patter our toes back and forth on the bleacher's footrest.

"What?" asks Caroline. "What did he say? Is it time for Wilson?"

"Almost Cabooh," Billy tells her.

And with that she yells, "Go Wilson! Go Wilson! You are the best bull rider and the best brother in the world. Go Wilson!"

This random outburst doesn't even bother Holly today.

We don't know the people here. We are all together to cheer for the big brother, united by an innate understanding of the treasure of this moment. This supreme connection takes center stage, putting our collective pain to rest.

We start to sway slightly together and sing along with Waylon and Willie, warning mamas not to let their babies become cowboys.

With each line, we sing louder, until the announcer interrupts and calls out the line-up. Wilson is sixth out of seven riders. After the fifth rider, we still don't have a winner, an eight-second rider. My eyes seek Wilson out. I find him, determination emanating from his tense body. As an older cowboy grabs his shoulders and barks one last pep talk, he puts in his mouthpiece and nods. With one effort, he scales the chute and lowers himself down over the raging beast. The trapped bull snorts, stomps, and bangs his shoulder into the barricade, trying to break the door with his horns. Balanced over him, Wilson runs his gloved hand up and down the rope, heating the rosin for stickiness. His forearm muscles are ripped and taut, veins bulging.

The sixth rider makes seven seconds. The announcer continues, "Okay, okay everybody. That was close, but no! Up next, we have a young rider to keep our eyes on. It's Wilson Heaton, from Watkinsville, Georgia. Let's see what this young cowboy can do."

We hold our breath and squeeze each other as Wilson tethers his left hand to the hot, sticky rope. He lowers his body down on top of the bull, leans out over the huge horns, and gives the official nod. The clock starts and the gate flings open. We stand and cheer like we're fans at the Super Bowl living out a bucket list moment.

The furious bull spins and flings his massive butt into the air. His feet thud back down as Wilson hangs on, one hand flying up in the air. He bucks again, front to back, front to back, and then he tries again to throw Wilson off by spinning in the other direction and bucking at once. It's six seconds in. Wilson starts to slide, but he uses the next leap into the air to pull back up to the center of the bull's back and grip again with his boots. And the horn blows!

"Ladies and gentlemen," the announcer bellows. "This young cowboy has done it. Congratulations, Wilson. You are the first bull rider to make eight seconds today!"

On the drive back home, the electricity in the car is palpable. Caroline can't contain her joy: "Wilson, you are the best bull rider in the world!"

He says, "Thanks, Caroline, but I'm not. I think the best bull rider who ever lived was Tuff Amos. One day, I will be legendary like Tuff Amos."

Holly bubbles with pride, too. "Wilson, I could see your hands slipping. I was screaming for you to hold on. I was like, 'Hold on, Wilson! Hold on!' And you did it!"

As the girls continue their praise, my mind wanders to a phone conversation I had with Holly. We gave her a cell phone for her birthday and I had become annoyed at how she would just sign off from calls with no warning or even a goodbye. She would just end the call as soon as the conversation no longer served her needs. So I called her out on it, explaining that you can't just hang up on people, and *especially* not your mother.

"Why do you do that?" I had asked. "You just end the call. No 'thank you,' no 'see ya later,' no 'I love you!'"

Without hesitation, she answered, "I just don't want to waste my minutes, Mom."

"Holly we have a family plan," I remind her. "It comes with unlimited minutes. You don't have to worry about that."

"No, Mom." Holly clarified, "I mean my *life minutes*. I don't want to waste my *life minutes*."

How did a 13-year-old girl come to treasure life minutes?

I think, *damn right, baby. Life minutes matter.* I have not yet stopped seizures from robbing Caroline of some of her life minutes. I see this as a warning and a responsibility. I must stop waiting for pain to evaporate because, like dandelion puffs, the chances for magic are blowing right by.

CHAPTER 15
THE PRETENDERS

It is clear—the wreckage of epilepsy is our new normal. It's a journey with no end in sight. To accept this doesn't mean I am powerless to it; I will never stop searching for a cure. But realizing it's a war and not a battle sends sparks through me. I now see what was once the mundane as opportunities to let magic blow in and make memories.

I'm cooking chili. But as I do, I shag dance with Wilson to *Domino* by Van Morrison. I swing Holly around as we belt out Shania Twain's *Man! I Feel Like a Woman*. As the chili simmers, we all move to the living room for some line dance shenanigans. Billy is the master. With his natural dance skills and his efforts as an elementary school teacher, he owns the Electric Slide. The kids are delighted. Miraculously, Caroline's memory kicks in and she joins us, with a smile on her face that is worth a million life minutes.

Later, as we finish dinner, Billy shares his big news. "Guess what? After next Thursday, no one can call me Ralphie ever again."

We all laugh, but Caroline is confused, "What? Who is Ralphie?"

Billy explains that Ralphie is a character in *A Christmas Story* who wears big, round glasses. This Thursday, Billy is getting Lasik surgery and he will no longer need glasses.

@

It's Thursday night and the surgery was seamless. I'm lying in my bed beside Caroline. She's sleeping soundly, and my eyes start to close when I hear Wilson call me. Now that's odd. I leap out of my bed and dart down the hall to his room.

"What's up, Honey? Are you okay?"

Silence. He says nothing.

"Wilson?" Still nothing, so I switch on the light. I ignore the sea of clothes, books, papers, and sports equipment that cover the carpet. I look right at Wilson's face and watch him try to speak. He struggles. I walk closer and sit on the foot of his bed. He doesn't sit up or even lift his head. His eyes dart from the ceiling to my knees, but they never meet my eyes.

I put my hand on his shin and say, "Breathe. Whatever it is, just breathe. We will figure it out together." I wait and continue, "Take your time. That's right. Just take some time and breathe."

He keeps trying to speak, but his lip quivers, his voice cracks, and the tears come again. I wait.

Finally, he whispers through tears, "Is. Dad. Gay?"

"What?" I am stunned.

He asks again with more courage, "Is my dad gay?"

"Wilson, I am married to him. I think I would know. No, he's not gay. Where ever did you get such an idea?"

The tears stop and anger steps in. "Just ask him. Go ask him. Right now. Go ask him. I heard him on the phone. I heard him."

I ask for more information, but he won't budge. "Please Mom. Just go ask him right now. Ask Dad if he's gay."

And so I do. I walk into Caroline's room where the streetlight lets me see Billy sleeping soundly in the old cherry twin bed. He is wearing the goggles that the Lasik surgery people gave him, making him look like an alien.

I walk over, sit at the foot of the bed and whisper, "Billy. Are you awake? Billy, wake up."

In classic Billy fashion, he bolts straight up in a scare, "What, what. What's wrong?" Calmly I say, "Billy, Wilson is very upset. He thinks you're gay. Something about a phone call he overheard. What in the hell is he talking about? He just kept insisting that I come in here right now and ask you myself."

Silence.

I try to see the husband I have known for almost two decades. But I can only see goggles and I think, *Alien. The unknown.*

I grip the bedspread, try to feel, to hold onto the life I think I know. But my grip is worthless. My world is about to slide again, like a boulder, down the wrong side of a mountain.

With still no response, I press on, "Billy? Billy. Are you gay?"

I can't see his eyes. I want to see his eyes, but I only see the damn alien goggles. His posture slumps. His shoulders start to shake as he sobs.

"You are gay?" I whisper.

I keep waiting. A few seconds. Maybe a minute. Maybe it's 10 minutes. I just know I am waiting, gripping the sheets, feeling the boulder teeter, about to slide.

Finally, he says, "I don't know. I think so. Maybe. Yes, I think so."

The boulder falls. It picks up unstoppable speed. I flash back to our very first date. I remember watching Billy's hand gestures when he got passionate. And I remember inspecting the way he had walked into the Golden Pantry to buy me a Tab. I thought, *Hm. Some of his gestures seem a little gay.* But I immediately admonished myself for being so stereotypically judgmental. And with that, I put it out of my head. Until now, almost 20 years later.

I wait for an explanation, for something more. But he just cries and says, "I love you. I have always loved you and I always will."

I trust him. I trust his words. "Do you think you just tried to push this away your whole life? Have you just lied to yourself? And it's finally to a point where you can't push it away anymore?"

He starts crying again. "Yes. I'm sorry. I'm so sorry. I would give anything to be the husband you deserve."

I stand up abruptly and say, "Well, I have to go back and talk to Wilson. I will make up some lie. He doesn't need to know about this right now. He can't handle what he's dealing with already. We can talk about this later."

I turn to walk out. I almost reach the door and then I turn back. "We will figure this out. Together. Okay?" He doesn't respond. "Billy, other than my mother, I trust you more than anyone I have ever known. You have never let me down. We will figure this out. I love you."

As I walk to leave again, I hear him choke back tears.

I walk straight back to Wilson's room believing that a lie will protect him.

"Wilson," I say firmly. "Your dad is not gay. Whatever you think you know or heard, it's a mistake. Everything is fine, okay? Your dad is the same dad you have always known. Can you please relax now and get some sleep?"

He says, "Okay. Thanks, Mom. I just needed to know." I kiss his cheek, his forehead, his cheek again, and I leave.

I'm not convinced he believes me. We both just pretend.

As I lie down again and stare up at the ceiling fan, I know I won't be sleeping tonight. Like an old movie, our wedding appears in my mind, followed by the births of each baby. Perhaps I should have known, or perhaps he wasn't always gay. Maybe I caused him to be turned off by women. I realize I am shocked. I'm shocked, but I'm not sad. A part of me feels relief. I know now that one day, someway, somehow, this marriage will end. And how awful is it that I think, *And it won't be all my fault?*

But the self-focused head talk stops as I look over at Caroline and think what she has endured in her young life. About Wilson and his inability to cope with emotional turmoil. About Holly and her protection of life minutes.

Life minutes can be rounded up into hours, days, and years. And life minutes can be broken down into seconds that can change your perspective on life forever. Two-minute-and-thirty-second cheer routines. Eight seconds on a bull. Ninety-second seizures. And tonight, two five-minute conversations jerked my life as I knew it and sent it speeding down the dark side of a mountain. But even the dark side of a mountain gets a few hours of sunlight. Once again, I feel the existence of light and darkness, hope and fear, simultaneously alive within me. Deep in my belly is a ripple of hope for me. For me, as a woman. Maybe, just maybe, I can find love again.

But for now, Billy and I focus solely on our children and decide we will just pretend.

CHAPTER 16
THE SHORT BUS

I walk into the kitchen, home from work a little early to find our caregiver Michelle at the sink. The tutor is settled at the breakfast table beside Caroline, who is hunched over a workbook with her head in her hand. The words on the page are *adapt, drastic, origin, persuade.* Her body is still and tense, the heat of determination permeating the room as she tries to learn these sixth-grade vocabulary words.

Michelle is emptying the dishwasher. She is a carefree college girl who believes that as long as she can pay her bills and pass her classes, she is in Athens, Georgia, to meet guys, celebrate friendships, and drink craft beer. Her long, graceful fingers are cradling a stack of plates as she greets me with her breezy smile and sun-kissed hair that dances long past her shoulders. She comes to our home, and lights it up with her charm and banter. I want to bottle her essence and diffuse it about our house like a sunshine fairy.

The tutor, Ms. Linda, sits erect yet at ease beside her student. She has thick, jet-black curly hair that glistens like brand-new, patent leather Mary Janes. Her eyes pour love through the royal blue readers perched on her nose. She was going to retire from teaching, but then decided that being a part-time tutor would be rewarding. I wonder if she feels rewarded right now. While Caroline makes it clear they've been focused on these words for far too long, Ms. Linda looks refreshed. With the words now covered, she says sweetly, "or - ih - gin." And she waits. She is completely devoted to these four fucking words. I cannot even begin to grasp the patience that this woman possesses.

As I hold my breath and wait, I flash back to Caroline's spelling bee prowess from the second grade, and my throat constricts. I quickly shake that memory off and try to absorb patience from Ms. Linda.

"O. R," Caroline begins. We keep waiting, hearing only the sound of Michelle stacking dishes in the cabinet. "O.R," she says again and then whispers, "or-ih-gin" to herself. Forks clink together as they are laid in their cubby. "O.R . . . . I. O.R.I.," she says and Ms. Linda smiles and nods. The silverware drawer clangs softly as it closes. I bite my lip. Caroline says, "O R. I. . . . . O.R.I.G.I.N."

I exhale. We all cheer, "Hooray! Yes! Way to go, Caroline!"

I dash upstairs, planning to change out of my linen suit, heels, and dangling earrings. As I put on my leggings and sneakers, my mind is still stuck on watching Caroline work so damn hard to learn four basic words. Three years ago, she would have known those words—three years ago when she was an actual sixth grader. I'm sitting on my bed, about to tie my shoe, when I stop and allow myself a moment of gratitude. I'm grateful because we finally moved her out of Oconee County High School. I imagine the torment that would have continued, the snickering and egregious jokes about her inability to keep up.

I think back to the day we took her to North Oconee High School, about six miles away. The people at the district office had agreed that she could attend the school she wasn't zoned for. They even offered to pick her up in the yellow mini-bus. You know the one. The short bus. The vehicle that inspired jokes that a less patient, less aware, less compassionate me may have laughed at. Today when I see a short bus, I see an intimate community of people who know how to live in the moment. It's a small bus filled with more fight, more unbiased love, and appreciation for friendship than would fill a mile-long train of normal-sized school buses.

There is nothing superior about North Oconee, except for Miss Faye, the school nurse who can make you feel safely wrapped in warm, pink taffy. We moved Caroline to the other high school in the county for one reason: bullying. It was relentless and its effects were compounding. Not more than a few days would go by without Caroline coming home in tears or Wilson getting into a fight defending his sister.

When she arrived at North Oconee, almost no one knew her. She was just a new girl who always had a personal paraprofessional with her and was in classes with other students who needed assistance. It's a relief that she is in a school where she is unaware of the ever-unattainable popular crowd. They aren't in her classes, and they aren't her friends. I had hopes that she would blend in, but that was a tad unrealistic.

She wasn't there even two weeks when the team of support staff decided she wouldn't be sitting at desks anymore. For each of her classes, they brought in a big, comfy chair much like you would find in your grandpa's den beside his pipe and WWII novels. They also gave her one of those lap desks with the beanbag underbelly to carry around. She could sit in the comfy chair and do her work on the little pink lap desk from Target. Unlike the traditional desk-chair unit, she couldn't flip this chair over from a seizure.

Schools still have a business to run. They have assets, like the athletes and star students. And then they have liabilities. Caroline is a liability. She cost them a new employee, fully devoted to her learning and safety, not to mention the new chairs, and finally a new bed in Miss Faye's clinic. They pushed for her to wear a helmet and remain in one classroom, in the same grandpa chair all day.

Billy and I pushed back. Her confidence is already damaged. The experience of being a ninth-grade girl posing as a grandpa who forgot to remove his bicycle helmet could be permanently detrimental. For now, we choose to take the risk. She is to stay off stairs, ledges, stools, and hot pavement. With the special accommodations and the attention from all new friendly faces, Caroline has a bit of a new lease on life.

I consider this a win as I walk back downstairs and ask Michelle about her weekend plans before she leaves. She says it's nothing much—a fraternity party, a mud-run, and something about a hookah lounge. Shortly after she and Ms. Linda drive away, I feel a familiar twinge. I feel envious of Linda's patience and Michelle's carefree spirit.

But as I imagine embracing the gifts of two other women, I realize, that's not me, that's not how I am built. I'm more fuel and fire. This makes me not envious, but grateful for the calm, billowy energy that Linda and Michelle bring into our lives. I will leave that to them, while I trust in my energy to keep fighting for Caroline.

Right now, I need the energy of how I approach life to deal with the five voicemails flashing from my phone. I can tell that four are from high schools that are my customers, and one is from Wilson's literature/homeroom teacher. I ask Caroline to arrange carrots and cucumber slices on a plate, knowing that will buy me some time. Without taking my eyes off her, I listen to the teacher's voicemail first. After I finish listening, I remain frozen, staring at my phone.

This moment of tension is interrupted when in walks the sun—Kathleen. She is still in her bright blue school nurse scrubs, carrying her insulated lunch sack. She looks at me and says, "My, how those rubies and pearls bring out the stains on your apron."

Still staring at my phone, I reach up and fumble with the forgotten earrings. She sits down beside Caroline and makes a joke about how her mom prefers her cucumbers whole. When she sees I don't even smirk, she inquires, "What's up? Maybe you could use one of these cucumbers."

"It's Wilson's teacher," I say. "Kathleen, something is wrong. He used to be this super-driven student. We actually used to beg him to stop worrying about school! That was his lit teacher. She said we are at the halfway mark for the semester, and he has not turned in one assignment. Nothing. He has a zero."

I sling my phone across the table at Kathleen and she looks at it.

"Damn Tara Belle, you better call these schools back. If you lose your clients, who's gonna buy your smokes?"

I let out a massive exhale and she continues, "We've got the cucumbers and the rest of this pathetic salad, don't we, Cabooh? Tell your mom to go out on the porch and call her customers before they get pissed."

I go out on the porch, but of course, before calling anyone back, I fire up my friendship with Marlboro Lights. Just as I exhale, I hear a car pull up. As I quickly put out the cigarette, I can hear Holly and Ellie. I wave the smoke off the porch as the voices get closer. Ellie is a college freshman and a true apostle of the Holy Bible. She is a leader in a big youth group at the mega church that convenes in downtown Athens. Unlike Michelle, Ellie is not attending UGA to make memories she may not remember. Ellie is devoted to bringing young people to God. Holly is one of these young people. Since Caroline's encephalitis, we have pretty much stopped attending church. So, when Ellie first walked into Holly's life, it seemed like a gift. But this new obsession with good and evil, with sin and redemption, has put enormous pressure on a little sixth-grade girl. Secretly,

Kathleen and I have nicknamed her Holy. Holy Holly.

The screen door flings open, Holly hurls her backpack onto the porch swing, and Ellie steps in behind her. Ellie's energy is bouncy. It matches her glossy brown hair, which always looks like it tumbled right out of a Clairol commercial for dazzling curls. She sports navy Keds and a bright red cardigan from the Gap. Her makeup is merely a trace of mascara behind trendy glasses. The wholesomeness is Hallmark gold. She attributes her effervescence to a love affair with Jesus. Amazing.

Ellie speaks first. "Oh, Miss Tara! The music had us all on fire. We could all feel Jesus with us. He cradled us with his love. We missed Caroline, though." She looks over at Holly, who is smiling, but only with her mouth. She continues, "Didn't we, Holly? We want Caroline with us. We will all protect her and take care of her. Right, Holly?"

Holly keeps smiling, but that's not how she smiles.

Ellie steps forward and hugs me. She smells like green apples and gardenias. I tell her Caroline is right inside and she is welcome to say hello. But she declines, "Oh, I wish! Mama is waiting for me. She made a big pot roast. Yum!" She rubs her flat stomach as she twirls around and darts away.

I wave with a smile, but I'm staring at Holly. She is sitting on the porch swing beside her massive backpack. With the toe of her shoe, she stabs at the ground, making the swing awkwardly oscillate against the beams behind it and back again. When the swing smacks the beams again, I get up to stop the destruction.

Holly's teary voice wells, "Just this once! Just this once I wanted to go and sing and pray. Without Caroline." Her chest heaves and exhales in little flutters as she continues. "But Ellie just guilts me. She told you that *we* want Caroline with us. That *we* will take care of her. *We* is *me*. She is always telling me she has to be there for all the kids and Caroline is my sister so I need to be there for her. Am I bad, Mom? Am I a bad sister? I don't want to go there and have to take care of Caroline. It makes me—" her voice trails to a breath, a heave, a gasp. "It makes me sad."

I want to sit down beside my little girl and make it all go away. I want to cradle her and take the pain, but I know I can't. If I shoulder her pain, I'm afraid I will melt into a puddle like Frosty the Snowman.

To absorb others' pain to a point of irreversible impact makes me think about my mom and how empathy was her greatest gift and most tragic trait. Her shoulders rarely relaxed, as if she were carrying the suffering of everyone she knew. She was never able to just let her worries take a knee.

I'm not my mom. I have never seen worry as fundamental to love; I see it as a self-inflicted barrier to living. I see how Caroline's challenges are affecting her brother and sister, but to let it translate to perpetual worry would paralyze me, allowing my flame to burn through my soul. Rather than worry, I seek fresh perspective. It's not only Caroline's journey that is impacting our family, but also my response to it. I have built this tough, protective shield around myself. I'm right here, and still, my kids miss their mom. I can't go back, but maybe I can minimize the scars.

My old familiar flame grounds me. I wrap my arms around Holly, pulling her to me as I stroke her head. And then I let go and stand tall. I dash out the porch screen door and start the Explorer. Holly yells at me, "Where are you going?"

"Just hold on," I say. I roll down all the windows, pop in the Judds' CD, crank it up, and come back to the porch. As I force Holly off the swing, a little smile emerges, starting from her eyes. *God, how I adore this kid.* I hand her the invisible microphone, and she can't resist. We start singing. We get louder and louder, dancing and looking at each other as if we think we are Naomi and Wynona.

Kathleen and Caroline come to the porch, but we don't stop. With arms linked, we share one imaginary microphone and squawk-sing our favorite lines with uninhibited commitment.

Later that night, I climb into my bed where Caroline is already asleep and think about the day. Caroline forgot how to spell words from the sixth grade; Wilson is on a dangerous path; and Holly is experiencing shame and feelings of neglect. As long as even one of my children is suffering, am I expected to reject the sun like a woman whose soul has turned to ash?

To do that, I would not have seen what else happened today. Today I saw Caroline experience the reward of not giving up. Kathleen reminded me that I'm not alone and that laughter is a holiday from heartache. I physically pulled Holly out of her hurt and into a moment of sheer glee.

Today hurt. And today was a win.

CHAPTER 17

YOU'RE SHITTIN' ME

We have been conditioned to not complain, to put on a happy face and be grateful because, our life could always be shittier. This is the trash talk that probably leads to eating, drinking, shopping, smoking, or screwing away our emotions. Heartache should not be disrespected; it should be acknowledged. It is only through feeling our heartache that we build a capacity for bigger, better, sweeter joy.

I'm seeing this, I know this, but living it takes some practice.

It's Friday afternoon and I arrive home at about 5:30. Walking through the kitchen and into the den, I find Billy sitting with the newspaper. Caroline is curled up with Bruiser, watching *Legally Blonde* for about the 400th time. I drop my keys on the counter and Billy looks up to greet me, "Hey, Tara. How did your leadership conference go? I'm sure you crushed it."

I agree that it was rewarding, and the school was really fired up about it. Then I ask, "Where are Holly and Wilson?"

"Wilson is at Jack's and Holly is at Julie's, both planning to spend the night." Billy folds the newspaper and gets up. We continue our tag-team duet. I'm headed up the stairs to change and he's headed out the door.

With Caroline quiet and safe on the floor with Bruiser, I slow my pace of taking off my suit and heels to pull on shorts and a tank top. Adjacent to my bedroom is an odd, tiny room, only as wide as a window and about nine feet long. It's probably meant for a bassinet, but it turned out to be the perfect place for my Total Gym. Yes, I have a Total Gym, the contraption that was one of the greatest infomercial success stories of all time. Christie Brinkley and Chuck Norris convinced millions that this single unit would transform their bodies and ultimately their lives. And then of course very few people ever actually used the damn thing. I, on the other hand, am one of those few people.

I love my Total Gym. The smooth pulley action soothes me. The power it takes to lift my body up and down the incline is an affirmation of my strength. And I can even use it for a cardio workout by moving fast on a low slope. I know you think smokers don't do cardio. Well again, a few of us do. It is part of my health routine. Well, it's part of my routine, because you certainly can't describe my habits as healthy.

When people ask me how I stay so thin, I quip, "Nothing but caffeine, nicotine, and Listerine until 2:30 every day." But that's not totally true; I like Scope. Monday through Friday mornings I am usually up by 5:00 and either out for a run or directly to the porch with my coffee and cigarette. After the chaos of getting teenagers up and committed to another day of school, I go directly to the Jittery Joe's drive-through. I enjoy another cup of coffee with my next cigarette as I drive to my first high school for the day. When I leave that high school, I will pop into the local gas station, buy a Diet Mountain Dew and enjoy that with yes, another smoke as I head to another high school.

We usually service schools during lunchtime, so by the time I'm packed up and off that campus, it's nearing 2:30. I'm ready to eat. My lunch is usually one of two options: Wendy's number six (spicy chicken sandwich with French fries, and a Diet Coke) or another Diet Mountain Dew accompanied by Lance cheese and peanut butter crackers and a Snicker's bar. So, in the evenings, I try to reward my body by cooking a healthy dinner and, if the morning didn't allow for it, some form of exercise: Enter kale, black-eyed peas, and the Total Gym.

Note: This is not a recommended weight management program for any woman who likes the idea of living long enough to see her last period or one of her kids pay a bill.

On this Friday afternoon, I plug in my iPod and prepare to tear up the Total Gym. I select a playlist of Prince, Rod Stewart, AC/DC, Alanis Morissette, 4 Non Blondes, and Janis Joplin. Listening to Janis Joplin croon about Bobby McGee smears happy onto my brain. What does she say about freedom? You can only have freedom when you have nothing left to lose. As much as this song fires up my soul, I realize I don't agree. Sorry Janis, RIP my sister.

I am learning about what freedom means to me. I think back to the day my kids learned of my best friend. Yep, they learned about my biggest shame, my cigarettes.

We were in California for Caroline's biofeedback experiment (what a crock of shit and thousands of dollars down the crapper that was). We were at the hotel getting ready to go out to eat. I hurried along so I could go down and smoke before we all left. I announced I was ready and would wait downstairs. Wilson, Caroline, and Holly all jumped at the chance to go down with me and dazzle strangers with their southern accents. I looked at those beaming faces and in that moment, I decided to be honest. I decided to stop trying to present perfection to my children.

"Well, I'm going outside. To have a cigarette," I announced boldly.

Wilson said he knew, but the girls were stunned. The questions and comments were very direct. I answered honestly about my shame, about how addicted I was, and how I feared if they knew, they too might choose to pick up a cigarette. My kids saw a new side of their mom that day. They saw me, a flawed human who is still striving to live more in line with her values. It was freeing. It was a small bite, but it whet my appetite for the freedom that comes from vulnerability.

I'm still on my Total Gym, lying on my belly. My shoulders and biceps pull my weight up the incline as I keep thinking about freedom. In contrast, slavery comes into my mind, the truest form of human captivity. Are today's ancestors of slaves even really free? Here we are, more than

150 years since the Civil War ended, and still, as I define freedom, few are free. There are still consequences today for people of color to fully own their truth. And then I see white, suburban people who have much less to fear from society put a veil over their truth. They tell their friends about the splendid perfection of their spouse, the latest feats of their gifted children, and their picturesque week-end of tailgating with corn hole, peach vodka, and buffalo chicken dip.

My hands are sweating, so I grip the handles harder and keep pulling my body up and down the slope. What is freedom, really? What are the ramifications of finding out? All these people who seem to live for college football and trips to Destin, Florida, I thought they were the free people. And perhaps, they are as free as they wish to be.

But not me. I'm not free.

I shield my truth every time I'm greeted with the clutch-and-tilt. I pretend to agree that God will fix Caroline right up when He decides the time has come. I don't lean into the genuine love and support that is being extended to me. I tell people I'm okay, *I'm fine.* Hell, I'm even pretending with Kathleen that Billy and I are still on a path to ever after. I have been wasting my fighting spirit on fighting off my truth and denying human connection.

After the 4 Non Blondes let me scream from the top of my lungs about what could be goin' on, I leave my tiny workout closet and head back downstairs. I text Kathleen and in a matter of minutes, she is in my kitchen, pulling two cold IPAs out of her insulated lunch sack. I peek at

Caroline again and decide to just let her sleep. I will deal with her being up all night later. I motion to Kathleen to be quiet and go sit on the porch.

We sit down, I pour the beer she brought into a glass and pull out my Marlboro Lights. I stare at Kathleen as I savor the ritual of selecting a single cigarette from a full pack, rotating my little pink lighter in my palm, rolling the gear to hear the click and smell the lighter fluid. She waits as I inhale and see the cigarette's tip burn a deep orange.

"You're still all sweaty from your Total Gym shit and you light a cigarette," she says, raising her glass, and with her signature sarcasm, nods as if my deadly habit is worthy of respect.

"I'm the master," I smile.

She keeps eyeing me as I watch my secondhand smoke fill the porch and seep into the backyard.

"What?" she asks. "What the fuck? You look weird."

I take another drag, exhale, and reply, "Have you ever thought that Billy might be gay?"

She stares for a second. "Well, no, I never thought Billy was gay. But when I first met you, I told Tracy Black that Tim and I were going to dinner with you and Billy. Tracy said she didn't know Billy was even married. She said she thought he was gay. So I informed Tracy of her ignorance. What's wrong? Y'all hit a dry spell?"

I tap my cigarette into the ashtray, cradle my beer and say, "Tracy was right."

I don't smile. I don't look away. I just search Kathleen's

eyes. The silence hangs in the air with the smoke. I get up, flip on the ceiling fan, sit back down, and think, *freedom.*

"Oh, come on. Stop fuckin' with me," she finally snips.

I keep staring at her as I bite into my bottom lip.

She settles in a bit and asks, "Can you give me a little more here, Tara Belle? Are you sure? How do you know? How long have you known?"

"Well," I begin, "for starters, I'm an idiot. I never even suspected it. But I do know this. Billy didn't fool me or deceive me. I know that without any doubt. He is just now admitting this to himself. But yes, I am sure. I've known for about a year."

With that, Kathleen stands up and steps toward me a bit, "A *year* ago! You're shittin' me. Come on. A year? And you're just now telling me? You have carried this around with you for 12 months, 365 days, and you never told me? Why didn't you tell me?"

I say nothing.

She tries again, "Who else knows?"

My eyes twinkle a little. I try to conceal my smile. "Billy."

She rolls her eyes and offers classic Kathleen comfort, "Well at least you have that vibrator you bought when you were in Atlanta a few years back."

I shake my head, "Nope. I got rid of it. Holly is always in my closet, so I was afraid she would find it." Grinning, I say, "As a matter of fact, I was afraid to throw it in the garbage, so I drove it to the corner and threw it in one of the trash cans at the Golden Pantry. I didn't even stop for gas or cigarettes."

Kathleen's eyes widen and laughter busts through the haze. At first, we both chuckle; our bellies contract and our chests leap in tandem. And then, the laughing becomes unstoppable. As I hold my gut, my eyes brim with tears. I am so filled with gratitude for this friendship, for this woman who gets me so fully, that I don't need to articulate anything more.

I finally catch my breath and wipe my eyes with the back of my hand. My smile relaxes as I say, "Don't be hurt, Kathleen. I was processing this. It has taken me a long time to grasp this. I wasn't hiding it from you; I was just keeping it for me until I could handle saying it out loud."

These unchained conversations with Kathleen give me oxygen. Over the next few weeks, Kathleen and I talk a lot about Billy and me. I realize I've spent the past year with my jaw tense and my shoulders slightly above the natural resting place.

I now sit tall from my sternum, walk a little bolder, smile a little broader. What once felt like shock has become a secret power. I don't feel regret. I don't feel shame.

I feel emboldened.

And, oddly, I feel gratitude. I think of the energy it took to pretend. I remember when Billy surprised me with a trip to New York, so many years ago. And a trip to the mountains to stay in a bed and breakfast. And even our last New Year's Eve as the pretend couple. We stayed at the Foundry in Athens and went to a Mother's Finest show. Just like New York and the mountains, we were trying to make it romantic, but it wasn't. Pretending is tiring, the opposite of freedom.

I love Billy, perhaps more than ever before. I think about all the years he gave me his very best. If I needed to work late or travel, he was always there, and never once complained. He did more than his fair share of cleaning, caring, planting, mowing, carpooling, and tutoring. His thoughtful, generous nature that showed me love daily cannot be erased. And now, we also have truth. Truth is a powerful bond.

I imagine that all these years, my mere presence was a symbolic reminder that he could not live as the man he desired to be. And yet, that was never projected onto me. During 19 years of marriage, I honestly can only remember one time that Billy said something to me that was not respectful. I remember it so clearly, because it stunned me. One Saturday afternoon, I walked in the front door and started nagging about something. I don't remember what. But I can still see him sit up on the couch, twist around to look at me, and say, "And I don't appreciate your bitchy-ass attitude." That's it. That is a direct quote. That is the collection of anything unkind or biting that Billy has ever said to me. As I write this, that still stands true today.

And now, it is my turn to serve Billy. I want to support him in finding his way. I want to be his best friend, his confidant, his biggest cheerleader. He is over 40 years old, and it is finally time for him to breathe fully, to wash away shame and guilt and to find connection in the way he was made to love. It's his time to live his truth, to be released into freedom.

CHAPTER 18
SHAKING AND ROCKING

As the sun begins to greet the morning, I'm finishing a run. My lungs beg for mercy while my legs long to leap. Something has grown inside me. It's not more fight. It's softer, like a perennial that promises to keep blooming no matter how harsh a winter she endures.

As I embrace my desire to love Billy in a new and generous way, my heart yearns to soar. I smile to myself as I look into the future. I see a family. A new kind of family.

It feels good to run before the world wakes up. Still breathless, I walk into the quiet house, pour myself a cup of coffee and head to the porch. As the steam escapes my mug and the smoke billows, my mood shifts, making space to let the dread seep in: another morning of poking, shaking, and yelling for Wilson to get out of the bed. He has only four weeks left of high school, but if he is absent again, he won't graduate.

As I climb the stairs, I can't help but consider how we got here. Where is my little boy, the intense perfectionist? At such a young age, Wilson had a propensity to try so hard and to love so deeply, you almost felt sorry for him. And now he's trapped, consumed with grief, but not able to look it in the eye. I know deep in my gut; he has been neglected. We ask for his help, knowing that he needs help himself. And so how has he responded? He helps. He does whatever we ask of him and then he runs. Now he's running at top speed away from a home where grief hovers, tears are inevitable, and peace is out of reach. Wilson won't express his feelings for fear of inflicting more pain on his family. So he drowns it out with a perpetual party.

I step out of the shower, throw on slacks and a blouse, head down the hallway, and open Wilson's bedroom door. I look around and see his life, passion, and chaos, littering a sea of dirty laundry. Coke bottles filled with tobacco spit, a bird's egg, a lighter, spurs, a Honey Bun wrapper, chaps, boots, condoms, a Dairy Queen cup, a snakeskin, and a bottle he uses to feed his pig at the high school agriculture barn. I see the book he has read countless times, *Where the Red Fern Grows* by Wilson Rawls. The 1961 novel is a tattered treasure, sitting under a cracked cell phone and an empty wallet.

I sit at the foot of his bed and recount the conversations we have had right here, and the countless times I have expressed my love and faith in him. His counselor insisted that ADHD medicine would be the help Wilson needed. As much I didn't want to drug another child, we tried it. Wilson hated it, said it made him depressed, unable to eat. The counselor also said she couldn't get him to open up, and until that happened, she couldn't help him.

I only see one other course of action. Not enforcing it feels like neglect, because I'm at least strong enough to see the truth. It's fear and weakness that stand in my way. I should take Wilson's keys, put a halt to his activities, and force him to stay home until he has a clean room, earns good grades, and gets up for school on his own. But I don't do this, because I'm afraid it will backfire. I'm too weak to inflict more suffering on my son.

If our home were peaceful, orderly, and not choking with the anticipation of the next eruption, perhaps I would have taken this step. Letting Wilson run free feels like neglect but confining him to the home that is the source of his suffering feels cruel. With his impulsive, intense nature, I fear it will cause him to run even harder, faster, until he makes a choice that has irreversible consequences. So I keep trying to coach, love, and support Wilson into a mature young man who can manage his heartache.

I lean down and kiss his cheek. As I expect, he doesn't move. I kiss him again, again, and again. I rub my hand over his head as my lip quivers. I start to bite my lip, but then resist, and let my body feel the hurt.

I whisper, "Wilson. Wilson. Please get up, Honey. Just today, please just get up."

Nothing.

As I start to shake him, I flashback to the morning of January 11, 2005. The morning I had tried to wake Caroline. Here I am again, about to shake my son, just like I did my daughter all those years ago. I will beg him to wake up, just like I begged her.

I wipe a tear from my lip and remember how many times I have told my kids about the power of the fighting spirit.

I start shaking Wilson and yelling, "Wilson, please, please, get up! You *cannot* miss another day of school. You have to graduate!"

And as I take a breath, to yell again, I hear it. A booming thud.

"No! My God! No!" I scream. "Somebody get up and help me! Billy, Holly! Get up! Get Wilson up! Caroline fell off my bed!"

The caffeine and nicotine, mixed with adrenaline and cortisol, shoot me down the hall in seconds. I skid into the floor, cradle Caroline's head and grow quiet. I hold my baby as the convulsions take me with them. Her lips turn blue as I use my forearm to protect her head from banging into the nightstand. As the shaking starts to ease, I gently blow in her face and search for injuries. First, I check her shoulder. She has already dislocated it twice, but it feels in place. Then I check her head. *Ooooh.* There it is. A goose egg. Because of the constant trauma that seizures are inflicting on her shoulder lately, as soon as she comes to, she will be writhing in pain.

I keep blowing and whisper, "It's okay, Honey. Mom is here. I'm right here. I'm so sorry, Honey. I'm just so, so sorry."

As I sit entwined with Caroline, gently rocking her, Holly appears in the doorway. "Is she okay, Mom?" she asks in a groggy voice. "What do you want me to do to help?"

"Get your brother up," I say, as I feel the cortisol elevate again.

She snaps, "No! Oh my God, Mom. No! When is he going to learn to get himself up? I get *my*self up. And I'm in seventh grade! I'm not getting him up. He's not my problem!"

That's the truth.

She storms back down the hallway and slams her bedroom door. As I rock Caroline, Holly continues her rant. She yells, "This sucks! Why is this our life? It sucks! I hate it!"

I keep sitting, rocking Caroline, and probably myself. I don't run, I don't scream back, I just let this be—a moment to let my heart ache.

CHAPTER 19
THE SANDWICH STAPLE

It's Friday night. Holly has a cheerleading competition in Columbus, Georgia, tomorrow, and we have to leave at 7:00 a.m. She is sitting at the kitchen counter, so I can coat small strands of her hair with Dippity Do and roll them in tiny, pink sponge curlers. It's a tedious job, but I enjoy it. I love playing with Holly's smooth, golden brown hair. And I enjoy the morning result when I pull the rollers out and scoop all the crunchy little curls into one bouncing ponytail. But even this simple pleasure has a new layer that stings. It's Caroline, sitting quietly, watching me do for Holly what I used to do for her. I remember to practice the acceptance of conflicting emotions, to feel the sting and still savor what is good in these few life minutes.

As much as I reject cheer culture, I love watching Holly perform on stage. The routines are short, only 150 seconds, but it's 150 seconds of happiness, a physiological boost to my spirits. I always hold onto Caroline, but for the entire routine, I don't look at her. I simply and fully delight in Holly and what she is able to do with her young body and untamed spirit.

There is an ass-load of preparation in front of this cheer mom before we can arrive in Columbus for 36 hours of waiting for the two and a half minutes of joy. The curlers are done. I'm busy packing anything and everything Caroline might need. I know, I know . . . all the other cheer moms are packing all the baubles, make up, uniforms, and snacks for their little darlings. But not Holly's mom. Holly has learned to do all this herself. Yes, the evil mom that I am, I actually let her do what she is capable of. She feels slighted by this. I wish I could say it's wisdom that told me to let Holly do for herself. But that's not it. It's simply an overloaded mom who needs her kid to do what she is able to do.

I wonder, *are self-sufficiency and motivation genetic, or are they the result of a lack of nurturing?* Holly has learned to make life happen for herself when I don't or can't agree to fill the role of mom to her satisfaction. I guess this trait could be inherited, but perhaps it's more of an environment repeating itself in a new generation. I still have vivid memories of learning to get myself where I wanted to go. The first was when I was six or seven years old, not older than seven, because we moved to South Carolina in the spring after my seventh birthday.

We were living in a Baltimore suburb where, at the end of the street, was an Episcopal church. My mom had taken us a time or two, but it was far from consistent. She was a night owl who struggled to get up in the morning, and my dad left early for golf. So, I decided to get myself to Sunday school. After a breakfast of Honeycombs and whole milk, I began the challenge of wriggling into thick white tights. The struggle was rewarded as I buttoned up a fancy dress made for twirling and buckled my feet into black patent leather shoes. They shimmered in the morning sun as I walked myself down the street to the church.

I knew how to find the second-grade classroom where little wooden chairs were tucked neatly under tables. The smell of glue and crayons lured me into my seat amid the bins that were organized with construction paper, pipe cleaners, and miniature scissors. The teacher was a young woman with flowing, silky brown hair and long fingernails painted in a rebellious green. Her earrings jangled softly as she placed Nilla Wafers onto paper napkins and poured Kool-Aid into tiny Dixie Cups after the prayer. I was captivated by the magical stories she read from the big Children's Bible.

It was only the end of Sunday school that I dreaded, which is probably why I remember it so clearly. When class was dismissed, I would take my tiny purse and my art project and pretend to do what all the other children did—look for my parents so we could go into the church service together. I stood on tiptoes and peered around crowds as if I were looking for my family, but when the other parents took their children's hands and walked into the sanctuary, I walked back home. Sundays were layered with both delight and loneliness.

This old familiar sandwich of dread and joy is becoming a menu staple for me. There is a part of the cheer competition I dread like never before. It's not because of the hundreds of glitter-covered princesses prancing about; it's watching Caroline watch all the girls do what she had worked so hard to be a part of. If I'm not physically holding onto her, I can't take my eyes off her, because of the threat of a seizure. But looking directly at her face, into her grim, wistful eyes feels like choosing to walk into a knife.

On those days, I resonate with something Billy and I have both said: She might be better off if she were worse off. I wish she couldn't remember ever being a cheerleader. I suspect that if her brain were even more damaged, she would be in less emotional agony. But that's not her reality. She remembers the past. She just can't seem to retain new information or make new memories. I feel grateful that Caroline's encephalitis didn't leave her with more significant challenges, but that cannot erase the heartache of how her memory tortures her.

The night has wound down; everyone is in bed except for me. I stare in the mirror before washing my face. As I rub the soap into my pores, I wonder if I am an anomaly, seeing life as layers of good stuff and sad shit.

Whether we see it this way or not, we all live sandwiched between heartache and happiness. More layers of happiness seem to be a universal objective, I suppose because that helps diminish the anguish life promises all of us. Perhaps the reason Holly is so self-sufficient is simply that she is chasing more of the good, racing away from the sad, just like her brother does. Recalling my promise to never relinquish the power of my spirit makes me believe that I too can layer in more happiness.

I daydream of more joy, dancing like a bird freed from its cage. I also dream of a strong, loving man who is creative and passionate and who treasures the simplest of gifts on this earth. Of course, I can't imagine any man signing up for a lifetime of what Caroline's slow decline will bring. But perhaps a boyfriend? I snicker internally, imagining someone who comes into my life for dates, weekend getaways, outdoor excursions, and mind-blowing sex. As I soothe my face with a final hot rinse, I realize with amazement that I have stopped talking myself out of these hopes. Climbing into bed beside Caroline, I keep letting myself dream of this love and how it could add more layers of joy to my life.

CHAPTER 20

NO BOYS ALLOWED

We made it. Wilson graduated. As I prepare for a small celebration at home, my head is filled with images of the three pairs of eyes I gazed into on the days they arrived in the world. Today, each image reminds me of their unique spirit. Holly's eyes are big, round, and golden brown. They greet you with unencumbered curiosity. Caroline's almond-shaped, Hershey-brown eyes reflect compassion. And Wilson has blue eyes, neither almond-shaped nor round. Wilson's eyes are deep-set. Penetrating. When they look at you, you know it. What strikes me on this day is that those piercing eyes are a perfect match to his graduation cap and gown.

Holly helps me decorate the kitchen with some photos that capture precious memories with Wilson, plus his senior portrait, a blue and white tablecloth, napkins, cake, banners, cards, and gifts.

The sound of his truck rumbles up the driveway. He walks out onto the back deck with his best buddy, Wade. Smiling with anticipation, he gives me a hug that is classic

Wilson. It's a hug that says, *"I'm here for you, Mom."* I love him for it. And I hate it. I don't want my son to feel the need to protect his mother. I want to light up his world, making him believe in himself, no matter what life throws his way.

I pull back from the hug and search his face. His eyes should be illuminated right now. But they won't look at me. I hold his cheeks in my hands until he finally glances into my eyes. I see a haze, a screen of gray and with that, release the face that transformed my understanding of love 18 years ago. I miss the eyes that tell each person they meet they are the most fascinating person in the room.

He pulls his blue and white tassel with the 2008 dangling emblem out of his front pocket and puts it in my hand.

"Will you keep this safe for me, Mom?" he asks.

Wilson and Wade eat a barbeque sandwich and a piece of cake in a matter of minutes. As if he senses the graduates are about to leave, Bruiser is pressing his entire body into Wilson's thigh, savoring each rub of Wilson's strong hand over his head and neck. I settle into the lawn chair, preparing to reminisce a bit, but almost instantly I hear raucous laughter and Eric Church blasting from speakers. Friends are waiting in the driveway.

Wilson jumps up, kisses me on the cheek, hugs his dad, tousles Holly's hair, and starts to hug Caroline.

She resists and reminds him, "Wilson, you said you would play the pencils at your happy graduation party."

Wilson stops, turns, looks at his sister, and tells Wade to tell the guys he needs five minutes. He fishes two pencils out of the junk drawer and settles down at the kitchen counter. Caroline's face lights up as Wilson makes a beat with his knuckles, elbows, the heels of his palms, and the pencils. The beat picks up and takes on a life of its own. Caroline beams. We all start to clap and dance like a scene out of *The Jerk* with Steve Martin.

But this joyful party scene lasts only about five minutes before he is ready to move on with his friends.

Wilson and Wade climb into an SUV full of new graduates. As they back out of the driveway, through my tears I see Wilson grinning, head bopping, playing the pencils on the dashboard.

In seven weeks, we will be moving Wilson into a dorm at Abraham Baldwin Agricultural College in Tifton, Georgia. I have seven more weeks to prove my son's ability to sleep normal hours, to clean his room, to get up for work, to control the partying. Seven more weeks of reminding him about the fighting spirit that is alive within him. Seven more weeks of pouring every ounce of heart and energy into preventing him from trashing his potential and wasting the rare magic of Wilson. Just seven more weeks. And then what? I try to believe that being away from a home that keeps wounds raw will be what Wilson needs to grow up and grow strong.

I'm driving home from work, zipping past the white picket fence-framed farms, blooming red and pink crepe myrtles, cows huddled under the shade of oak trees. I'm squeezing the steering wheel, so deep in thought I don't even remember to light a cigarette and take in the early summer glory of north Georgia. My heart pounds in my ears as my mind ricochets from the growing desire for Billy to just go and be out of the house, and the fear around the fact that Wilson is the one who is leaving.

The thick threads of the steering wheel are burrowing into my fingers. I loosen my grip, reach for my little pink lighter and click it against the top of my Diet Mountain Dew. *Maybe Wilson will just Dew it*, I chuckle. But deep in my gut, I know we are not a Mountain Dew commercial. My insides burn with an apocalyptic warning. Even so, I know I will go through the motions, planning and preparing just like the other parents of the 377 graduates in his class. We will check every item off the college-ready list and countdown to that emotional day of moving in. I think I'm supposed to cry. Everyone cries. I could try to cry, but I suspect I have cried the quota of tears you are allotted in life. Did I not properly ration my tears? My lifetime allocation has been spent and I don't have any left to shed for what epilepsy and my obsession with beating it have done to my oldest child, my baby girl, and to a marriage that is now a roommate agreement.

Billy and I decided we would live as friends for now. We would say nothing to the kids and keep up our tag-team charade. But lately, it's not a team. It's a mom with three kids, plus this emotionally absent guy who lives in one of the bedrooms and helps in any way I ask. When I work late or have a business trip, Billy steps up and takes care of everything. But when I'm at home, well, he isn't. He is gone and I never really know where.

I remember last December, he left one Saturday morning and said he was going Christmas shopping all day in Atlanta. By the time he got back home, I was asleep. Days later at his family's Christmas gathering and again on Christmas morning, the wares from his shopping trip were revealed and they all had one thing in common: Brookstone. That's right. He had driven the 65 miles to Atlanta, spent an entire day and evening, and returned with all of his purchases from one single store inside Lenox Mall. To this day, I can't see a personal massaging gadget or digital photo frame without flashing back to the Christmas of 2007. But in this moment, Brookstone offers a glaring message—we are not a team.

"This is bullshit," I say out loud to no one as I hit the breaks for the one stop sign in Ila, Georgia. I thought we were going to be a family. At first, I was energized by our arrangement. The weight of pretending to be in romantic love had been released. I sprouted wings and could flutter again. During my morning runs or Total Gym routines, I let my mind wander with hope to a day when I would perhaps have love again. Exercising while imagining love pumped happy chemicals into my brain and gave me a glorious energy. That energy was my fuel for a while. But to have hope without action eventually becomes only a fairy tale.

Why are we doing this? I know we are not fooling our children. Is this the message I want to send to them—that we must sacrifice ourselves and live with the burden of projecting happiness to the world? I know the answer. I want to model truth and self-worth. I can't keep waiting to win the war on seizures before I start to take back my life.

I'm putting an end to this siloed arrangement, I promise myself.

When I decide something, it releases me. Angst is not manifested through action; it tortures me during the assessing and obsessing that lead to the action. Once I choose what to do and how to do it, the turmoil dissipates. So, as I speed onto the ramp toward home, I decide. I'm not going to keep living in a marriage that is lonelier than being alone. As long as we live like roommates, there is no hope of being anything but somatically forsaken. I would remain this lonely mom who lives in the shadows of the woman she desires to be.

I don't stop at the office. I drive straight home, thrust my Explorer into park, and charge into the house. As I gulp in air, Billy is already rising to leave, but I protest.

"Are you in a hurry?" I ask. Before he can answer, I say, "We should talk."

We both glance at Caroline sleeping peacefully on the floor with Bruiser and we head out to the porch in silence.

I begin with, "Billy, I love you. I am so sorry for what you are dealing with. But the thing is, I'm not sure our arrangement is going to work out any longer."

He waits.

I continue, "When we decided to stay together for now, I thought we were going to actually be more of a family. But we aren't. It feels like you are uninvested. Yes, you're always here when we need you. But other than that, it's like you just live here. You and I both know you are only going through the motions and your head is somewhere else. I don't want to live like this. I want you to be a part of this family. I want you here and with me, managing this shit storm together. You leave every chance you get. I don't really know where you go or who you are with, but I'm asking you to stop."

Silence. Billy's head is down, his shoulders drooped. Without even looking up he says, "And what if I can't?"

I force out the words, "Then I want you to leave."

It's only three more weeks until Wilson moves into the dorms. Billy and I are sitting on the porch, him with his Bud Light, me with my Marlboro Light. We are sitting where we always sit. He is on the swing he loves, the one we gave him for Father's Day the year we moved into this house. I smile, remembering Wilson and his cousin working so hard to hang it. I'm sitting in my usual chair, the one beside the old pine bar cart that hides the ashtray. We are waiting for Wilson.

"He said he would be home by six," I say to Billy as he nervously fidgets with his beer bottle. Oddly, I find myself wondering, do gay guys drink Bud Light? And obsess over college football? Those don't seem like gay things. I thought gay guys drank sangria or Cosmopolitans and went to the theater.

I want to lighten the mood on this heavy porch, so I try to make Billy smile with my ridiculous stereotyping. "Billy, do gay guys drink Bud Light? I mean, shouldn't you be drinking something a bit more, you know, *boujee*?"

Billy laughs with a "Bah! I don't give a fuck what they drink. I've been drinking Bud Light since I was eighteen years old. When I die, I hope it's with an ice-cold Bud Light in my hand and scorching chicken wing sauce on my lips."

"Are you sure you're gay?" I ask with a grin, although I'm also checking to make sure I didn't cause it. I wonder if I somehow became so unappealing to Billy over the years that he was not only turned off by me, but by all women.

"I mean, maybe it's me," I say. "Maybe you are just no longer attracted to me. This delicious, hot piece of ass sitting across from you, that clearly any man would give his right testicle to fuck." I laugh. "Maybe you don't like my particular type, but you may want another type of woman. The sweet, tiny, quiet kind of woman who is home from work by five, decorates for all the holidays, and follows all the rules. Seriously, maybe you're not gay. Maybe you just don't want to be with me. And because I'm so damn hot, you think you might be gay." I flash a giant, laughing grin.

Billy sets down his beer bottle and laughs with one loud clap. "Ha! Tara! Ha!" He laughs again. "First of all, you have never needed to decorate, because I do it. Secondly, thank God for your rule-breaking ways. Where would Caroline be without it? Where would your career be if you followed the status quo? And third of all, you are the most beautiful woman I have ever known. And yes, I am sure. For you, for our family, I wish I was not made this way. But I am. I am definitely gay."

We hear Wilson's truck roar up the driveway. I put away the cigarette that I was about to light. The garage door is closed, forcing him to come in through the screened porch where we are sitting.

"Hey, what's up," he says as he heads toward the kitchen.

"Wilson," I say. "I told you we want to talk to you. Please sit down." He calls for Bruiser, brings him onto the porch to pet, and sits down.

I look at Billy. I realize we didn't rehearse this.

Thankfully, Billy begins, "Wilson, your mom and I love each other very much. We love you kids more than anything on this earth. But, well, we have decided to separate."

Silence.

"Not much will change, especially for you," Billy says. "We will still have holidays together, be together a lot, but I am moving out in a few weeks."

We wait.

"Are you getting a divorce?" Wilson asks.

"Yes, we are." I answer before Billy tries to sugar coat it.

"Well, if this makes y'all happy, then that's all that matters," Wilson states solemnly.

I try to find his eyes, but per his usual lately, they elude me and remain fixed on Bruiser.

Finally, he looks up, but away from us and out into the back yard. Quietly he asks, "So what now? Are you selling the house?"

"Your dad is moving into an apartment in downtown Athens in two weeks," I tell him. "We will stay right here."

"All alone?" Wilson asks his dad.

"Me and Bru-man," Billy says. "I'm taking Bruiser with me."

"Is that everything?" Wilson asks, still staring into the yard.

"Well, yes," I say. "But I thought you might have questions, concerns, need to talk about it."

Wilson stands up and says, "No. I'm fine. Thanks for telling me. Do Caroline and Holly know?"

"Not yet," I say. "We will tell them tomorrow after Holly gets home from cheerleading camp." Wilson walks into the house, leaving Bruiser whimpering after him at the door.

Billy reaches for his Bud Light and I pull the ashtray back out from under the old bar cart. I light. He swigs. He swings. I exhale. I see the toxic smoke permeate the porch. I get up, flip on the fan, and sit back down with my best friend clamped between two fingers. Billy's eyes fill with tears. His chest breathes with a tremor as he takes the back of his free hand and wipes away the tears that escaped his eyes. He makes that sound from the top of his throat when he can't find words but needs a release, "Uuuuhhhhhhh!"

The hurt in Billy's face causes me to tell him, "Billy, this isn't an ending. It's a new beginning for us, to be close in a way that we have never known. I'm proud of you for facing your truth. But I know it's just the beginning of a tumultuous discovering." He starts to cry.

"You might get some hot-ass boyfriend, Billy Heaton, but I'm always going to be your best friend. Do you hear me? I love you. I want a new friendship to grow. And I think that can happen. After you move out." I slide the overflowing ashtray back under the cart and walk into the house. A single mom's house. My house.

We are once again on the porch. Billy and I, in our same positions, but with Caroline and Holly on the little loveseat. Billy has just finished the same speech he gave Wilson two days ago. Watching Caroline's lips tremble and Holly's eyes fill with tears make me want to take it back. This is the moment that keeps unhappy couples together. The soul-gripping heartache of saying to your innocent kids, "We are getting a divorce."

Caroline speaks first through her tears, "Dad. No. No. No, you are not leaving. No!"

And Holly chimes in, "This is the worst thing in my life. Everything we have been through and now my parents are breaking up! This is not fair!"

I try to comfort them, but the crying is inconsolable. Holly finally composes herself enough to open her phone. She dials and begins to sob into the phone, "Ellie! Ellie, can you please come get me? I have to leave. My parents . . . My parents just told me they are getting, getting . . . getting DIVORCED!"

"I'm coming too," Caroline says.

Holly looks at me with disgust, grabs Caroline's hand and bolts down the driveway. From the dining room window, I watch Holly dig her heel into our lawn and Caroline sit in the grass with her face in her hands as they wait for their savior to arrive. My girls welcome the hugs from Miss

Ellie of Sunnybrook Farm. Holly jumps in the front seat, Caroline, without objection, climbs into the back and they are gone.

It's move-in day at Wilson's college, so Billy, Caroline, and I follow Wilson to Tifton. We have done all the things. We checked off every item. He has new sheets. They match. He has a bucket to carry his soap and toothbrush to the shower. He has a hamper and a drawstring laundry bag. He has all new socks. They match, too. So, yep. He has everything he needs to win at college.

I try to help organize drawers and suggest we make a Target run for some last-minute items. But Wilson has no interest in setting up his room. He prefers to get out and meet new people. He will find the people with palpable energy and an insatiable zest for living their life minutes to capacity.

This day is not the dreamy, teary, proud moment many parents imagine. In my head, I can hear other parents telling their sons, "We have given you our best. You have all you need to be successful." But I can't say that. I gave Wilson all I could, but it was far from my best.

Billy hugs Wilson and tells him he believes in him. I smooch his cheeks, hug him tightly, and half-beg him to take care of himself. Caroline tells him that she will miss riding in his truck, even if it is messier than his room. And, of course, she tells him he is the best brother in the world. His lips stiffen, trying not to let them quiver as he hugs his sister. There is nothing more to say or offer in pursuit of success. Driving away, I try to remain steady, knowing we are headed back to one more day of moving out.

Billy is preparing to drive off for the last time and sleep in his new apartment. I don't look at him. I kneel down and hold Bruiser's face. As I kiss that soft little space between his ears, I remember how worried I was that he would jump on Caroline when she got home from the hospital for the first time. But he didn't. Somehow, he knew she was fragile. He just sat beside her as if it were his time to protect her. And I remember the one time he growled and tried to bite someone. It was Laney. She had stopped by the house to get one of her CDs out of Caroline's room. But Bruiser felt it. He knew his family had pure anger toward this child, because she was the queen mean girl from Caroline's old high school. Now, I rub his neck, his back, and I throw my arms around him. I pull back and say, "Kiss, Bruiser. Give kiss." He bumps his lips to mine, as I trained him to do.

I stand up, keeping my hand on his soft, familiar head, and try to lighten the air. "Wait, Billy. This is some bullshit. You got to take Bruiser and I'm stuck here with both girls? Can we trade? I will trade you Caroline for Bruiser." Billy chuckles out that familiar laugh through tears.

So I say, "Okay, or Holly. You can have Holly."

We smile. We hug. He says, "Come on, Bru-man." And they walk out the door. Without looking up, Billy closes it for the last time—the first time he won't be returning through that door to his home.

That night, with Wilson and Billy both gone, I lie in my bed feeling the emptiness in the house. It's just us girls. I consider what gives kids the best chance for winning at life. What is the ideal foundation for delivering a responsible, confident human to the world? I think it's something my kids can barely remember having—a safe place to land at the end of the day. I haven't given that to my children. From the start, I knew I wanted them to walk into the kitchen and feel the energy of love and of joy. I wanted to give them solid footing, happy memories, a safe place to lay their sweet heads at night.

But ever since January 11, 2005, they have not had a comforting space called home. They have lived in fear of the next crash. Another seizure. Another blow from a failed therapy, drug, or procedure. Will Mom be yelling into the phone at a doctor or a teacher? Will Dad be raging about how Caroline has been treated by her old classmates? Will we all be screaming for Wilson to get out of bed? Will Holly shout or wallow just to be heard? Will Caroline wail "Why me?" again and again?

In most of these cases, I can't prevent the crashing, but I can change how I respond. *That* I have power over. I fire up my determination and will myself to absorb the energy of the next crash. Rather than fighting it off, I will use it. I will transform it and set it free to bring light to someone else's world.

CHAPTER 21
HOLY HOLLY

"Mom! Mom, can I go to Africa?" Holly asks as she bursts into the kitchen, flings her mint-green backpack across the tile floor, and hops up to the counter. I pick up a few cucumber slices, hand them to her and continue slicing.

"Jesus, Holly. The divorce isn't that bad. You don't need to go to Africa," I say with a smile.

But she doesn't focus on the joke. She says, "Please don't use Jesus's name in vain. I don't want to go to Africa forever. It's a mission trip! Please can I go?"

She keeps talking about this mission trip in true Holly fashion. She sits up straight, bobbling her head and talking with her hands. Light shines from her eyes.

The magic energy of this kid fills me and pours back out in the form of a rhythmic, celery-chopping dance. I look up at her eyes, not really listening to what she is saying, but just absorbing the melody of her voice.

She snatches a few more cucumber slices from the bowl as my mind wanders back to when I had picked up my chattering second-grader from school. We drove off as Holly bobbled and discussed the day as if it were the most important day in her life. She unfolded her perspective on the teacher's strategy and how it affected each student. She finally wound down with a question, asking me what I thought.

But my response was not an answer to her question. Unfiltered admiration for my seven-year-old daughter bubbled out of me with the words, "I simply *adore* you!"

She shot back with a literal hair toss, "Um, excuse me?"

"Oh, I do! Holly Pauline, I simply *adore* you! You light up my world. You make me want to dance and sing and celebrate with all my might. I simply—"

And she finished my sentence with a dramatic Zsa Zsa Gabor-esque, "*adooore* you."

From that day forward, it became our own little mantra. In this moment, I can feel it still alive within me, and in her.

With wooden tongs, my hands lead a dance through the salad while Holly winds down from the African mission trip sales presentation. Again, she is talking as if it's the most important day of her life. But isn't it? Isn't today the most important of her life? Certainly, today is just another Tuesday, and today is a celebration of a complex, emotionally charged young girl. These are life minutes, baby. I think, *of course you can fucking go to Africa. With that ferocious spirit, with that ability to take hold of life minutes, oh yeah, go!*

"Well mom? Can I go?" She waits.

I freeze the salad tongs and look at those round, golden browns. From my soul, I smile back at her and say, "I simply—"

Like the Dalai Lama, she spreads her arms open to the world and completes the sentiment "*adooore* you."

Our house of chaos has tempered quite a bit. Caroline is on a new diet that has her seizures much less severe and less frequent. And with Wilson away at college and Billy just around the corner, we are finding some peace.

I'm sitting at my office desk, methodically working my way through a stack of paperwork. I might be the boss in here, but thankfully my office manager Dena tells me exactly what I need to do. I wonder what the hell I would do without her. She keeps this ship afloat no matter what I seem to face. She gives me all the customer problems, product issues, and client challenges. I just power through. It's what I do.

Dena appears at my office door. "Wilson is on the phone. He tried your cell, but didn't reach you. He's on line two. Sounds urgent," she says with a look that feels like pity splashing down on me.

Fuuuck, I think as I snatch up the phone. "Wilson? What's wrong?"

Isn't it weird how you can hear your kid cry even when he is silent? I bite my bottom lip, grip the phone cord.

He finally says, "Mom!"

More silence as I bite harder, imagining a wreck or worse.

"I'm sorry. I'm so sorry, but I think I'm not going to pass any of my classes. I just had to tell you. I've tried to figure this out, but I think it's too late."

As he rambles, I think about what I have tried to teach and to model to my children. The minute I blame failure on anyone other than myself, I become powerless. I must take action. Action is how I keep hope alive. I have to believe I have also passed that on to Wilson. It's his time to take action.

"Wilson," I say calmly. "You call me every week, screaming into the phone about a lost wallet, a broken alarm clock, a fight. You lost your truck, you don't have money, you can't do laundry. And the list goes on. You will be on probation after one semester. That means you have one more semester to figure this out. I will help you however I can. But from where I sit, you need to learn to stop partying and start the work of life. Or you won't survive. With all my heart, I love you. I believe in you." And I hang up the phone.

Rather than look for a reason to leave and have a cigarette, I stare at Dena as she works on a marketing flyer. I wonder how she would have responded if that were her kid calling to say they are blowing up their future, one beer at a time. I don't really have to wonder. She would get up, clock out, pack a bag, and be on the road to save her child. But I don't know how to save a young man who insists he doesn't need help. I think about Holly and how she seems to figure things out for herself when I don't come running. Maybe telling Wilson that I trust he can figure this out is what he needs. My decision gives me a moment of calm and so I reach for the phone to return a call to an upset customer.

But before I finish dialing, Dena appears in the doorway again. Her compassion has materialized into tears. She doesn't even ask about Wilson. She just kind of chokes out, "Michelle just called. She said you need to get home fast. Caroline is hurt."

Dena tries to continue, but I just grab my keys, kiss her cheek, and leave.

I slam the Explorer into park in the driveway, run through the garage, and into the kitchen.

Michelle is sitting on the kitchen floor with Caroline's head in her lap. She holds a blood-soaked towel under Caroline's chin.

"I'm so sorry, Miss Tara," Michelle begins. "I know she shouldn't sit on the barstools. But I was right beside her! She just slammed to the ground and started seizing. I . . . I couldn't catch her. It was so fast. And it wasn't like her other seizures. Her whole body . . . Her whole body was jerking. I mean really hard." She looks up at me with an ashen face and red-rimmed eyelids. "I think she needs stitches."

I peek under the towel. "Oh yeah. Let's get you to the hospital, Caroline. We need to fix that gash."

As Michelle helps me stand her up, I question the seizure. My heart is taking another disappointing blow. "Caroline, did you eat anything today you weren't supposed to? Did you eat any sugar, or bread, or maybe drink someone's drink that you thought was your water?"

Caroline looks at me with a slightly drooping, but furrowed brow, and in slurred speech asks, "Whuths's a gash?"

I assure Michelle that this isn't her fault. "Everything we try runs its course, Honey. This isn't on you. I have been letting her sit there some, too."

It has been months since she had one of these tonic-clonic seizures that come without the warning of an aura. I just hope she screwed up our latest attempt at seizure control through diet: no sugar, no gluten, no dairy. But deep down, I doubt it. I really think this has run its course and we are about to be on another journey in search of new answers.

CHAPTER 22
SUSHI AND A GERMAN

Caroline and Holly have gone to bed, and I have been researching the latest trials for intractable epilepsy secondary to viral infection. When I can't stare at the screen any longer, I file my notes, go out to the porch and sit with my cigarettes. But before lighting one, I just listen. The wind whistles softly as the occasional car whirs past.

I wonder if the people in the cars are heading home to simple pleasantries and predictable lives. I think about Caroline, what she has lost, and about this desperation I have to stop the seizures and give her some joy. The seizures are not only taking moments from Caroline in real time, but they are stealing her memory. She remembers what happened years ago, but unless something extremely emotional took place, she doesn't remember last week.

I hope she never forgets Jamaica. It was her sixteenth birthday gift. Since she couldn't get a driver's license like every other 16-year-old, I wanted to take her on a trip. I thought a trip would be healing for both of my girls. The stress of Caroline's confusion, depression, and safety were still front and center.

Add to that, my concern about Holly's obsession with Jesus was mounting. She was always an anxious child, worrying about anything from kidnappers to germs. But now she lives with this consuming belief that she must try harder to understand and accept God's almighty master plan. She has to identify all her sins and remember to pray for forgiveness, or she will end up in eternity with the Devil himself. Not only did I hope this trip would make a memory of joy for Caroline, but I hoped it would give my 13-year-old girl a break from living under the constant weight of the Bible.

For the birthday trip, I had told Caroline she could choose to go anywhere she wanted. She chose Australia. Okay, so I lied. Jamaica was a close second. It was a girls' trip. Kathleen, Holly, Caroline and I went to a *luxury resort* that was definitely not luxury. But the oddities of the not-so-luxurious resort added to the laughter and the makings of memories.

When we took off for Jamaica, I tried to show my girls that we are not barred from joy. I focused on intention, on making the most of life minutes, and joy won.

I remember the reaction from almost every Jamaican person who witnessed one of Caroline's seizures. They all had the same prescription, which consisted of Plan A and Plan B. Plan A was, "Oh, she has de fits. She needs some ganja, man. You want, I can get you some ganja. Can she smoke, man?"

At this moment, I would look over at Kathleen and then Holly. Kathleen answered first, "Um no, man. She can't smoke. But I can."

And then Holy Holly would object, "Mom! No! You better not buy marijuana! We could go to jail! No!"

Each time I assured her we would not be making any drug deals.

And then the confident Jamaican had Plan B, "Den give her da shoe. Ya man. Put a shoe over her face when she has de fits. Eet will stop dem."

I kept questioning this remedy with disbelief. "Put a shoe over her face? Come on now." But the native always insisted, "Ya man. It just has to be her shoe. If she has a fit, put de shoe over her face. She will come out of it like straight away."

We all giggled at this.

The girls were happy and free. I remember my joy in Jamaica, too. Kathleen and I always woke up much earlier than Caroline and Holly. We took our coffee to the pool deck and read Chelsea Handler's books, *My Horizontal Life* and *Are You There, Vodka? It's me, Chelsea*. We read in silence until one of us uncovered a nugget that had to be shared. The passage was read aloud and then we would laugh like two delirious 12-year-old girls who had been up all night eating candy and making prank phone calls. I bet anyone who sauntered by thought we were certainly smoking the ganja. Eventually, we packed up the books and took our caffeine-endorphin buzz back to the room to get the girls up and start the day.

The week flew by. We went on excursions every morning, lay in the sun in the afternoon, and then, before dinner, we always found ourselves playing billiards in our swimsuits. It was easy fun. The seizures had been mild, Holly seemed happy when she forgot to worry, and having Kathleen there kept me feeling not alone and anticipating laughter.

On the last night, we attended the resort's final event—a big dance party. Dancing, something Caroline, Holly, and I all love to do. The banquet hall-turned dance floor was pulsing with beats from the eighties to the present.

I thought, if Caroline gets too hot or out of breath, she will have a seizure for sure. That's a fact. But right now, she is having fun. Real fun. We are going to own this moment carefree. I danced with a smile so big it could crack my face. My girls' smiles felt like rainbow sprinkles on my skin. When I locked eyes with Kathleen, I saw a smile that made love so simple. She saw her friend let pain sit its ass down and make room for joy.

No one mentioned leaving the dance early or taking it easy. We just knew it was time to dance. By the time they played the last song, we were covered in sweat. Full of energy and laughter, we walked back to our room. I held onto Caroline as we climbed the stairs and walked to our door. Right as Kathleen was fumbling with the key, Caroline crashed down. I took the fall with her and cradled her head, protecting her from banging into the stucco wall.

The familiar reality of helplessness slapped into me as I yelled at Kathleen, "Give me that fucking shoe!"

She grabbed Caroline's flip-flop and handed it to me. I smashed it down over Caroline's face and waited to witness a Jamaican miracle. She kept seizing, I kept holding the shoe.

When the seizure subsided, we were able to get Caroline safely inside and resting comfortably on the bed. We sat quietly, catching our breath and letting the range of emotions from the past three hours gel.

Kathleen broke the silence. "Give me that fucking shoe!" she barked. And the laughter erupted, even from Holly.

I finally defended myself, "Hey. It was worth a shot!"

To this day, when Kathleen sees my stress rise, she can derail it by simply spewing, "Give me that fucking shoe!"

Now as I sit here on the porch at home, the beauty of this memory pours over me, reminding me I'm not banned from happiness. I will not hold out for the absence of pain as if it's a permission slip for joy. I could wait a lifetime. The pain, it's here to stay. But that doesn't mean I'm eternally tethered to it. It lives in me, where I can use it as fuel to gift joy back out into the world. Maybe one day, when people ask me where I get my energy, I won't respond with, "caffeine, nicotine, and Listerine." I will tell them it's a focus on the acceptance of pain and the intention of joy.

My breath is easy as I stare out into the dark night. My cell phone rings. It's my client who has become my friend.

"Hey, Chipper," I say into the phone with a smile.

"Hey Tara Belle," he says, wasting no time getting to the purpose of his call. "I know you said you weren't ready to meet anyone. But I'm just asking again. I really want you to meet my neighbor. He's going through a divorce, too. He's kinda quiet. He stays in shape. He walks a lot. He's an engineer. He's from Germany. He's cool. Oh, and he doesn't drink."

Silence.

"Tara Belle?"

I smile. "Fine."

"No shit? You'll meet him?"

"Chipper," I say with a giggle. "Let me get this straight. You think that a quiet, sober, German engineer who takes a lot of walks is a guy for me? Is he a recovering alcoholic? Is he uber religious? What's his story?"

It's Friday, November 19, 2008. We have agreed on a double date at Shokitini, the new sushi restaurant in Athens. Billy is with the girls and I'm driving to Chipper's house to meet this sober German engineer. Chipper has told me three times that this guy named Mike is in good shape. I deduce that Herr Mike must be unfortunate as far as facial features go. But hell, it's one evening. Even so, I feel nervous. This is a date, I guess. A date. Poor dude. I hope he doesn't want to get close to me. Think of the shit show he would be unwittingly signing up for.

Maybe I should ask him to sign a waiver before he dabs the first tuna roll into his soy sauce. The waiver would state: *I, Herr Mike, am of sound mind and body. I enter into this meeting fully aware of the potential for disaster, trauma, and emotional chaos. I will not hold anyone but myself liable for the inevitable damages in my future, resulting from my choosing to enter into a relationship with Tara Heaton.*

I chuckle at the thought. I know, no one of sound mind and body would willingly succumb to loving a woman whose life rides like an off-roading ATV.

As I pull into the driveway, Chipper's wife walks out to greet me. "Hey, girl. Oh, you look, um, like you're going to work. Oh, you look pretty, but just well, a turtleneck sweater and dress pants?"

"Well, shit, Cheryl, I haven't been on a date, or even out past 8 p.m. in a long time. My miniskirts are a little dusty."

She grabs my arm and as we walk into her living room, she whispers, "I think he's nervous."

Chipper greets me as if this is just some ordinary Friday. "Hey, Tara Belle, come on in."

I look across the room and see a guy dressed in jeans, a white oxford shirt, and a gray, wool flat cap. I walk over in my work clothes and like a dope, greet him in my work persona. I hold out my hand to shake his and say, "Hi, I'm Tara Heaton."

He shakes my hand and Chipper says, "Mikey, take that hat off."

As Mike reaches up to take off the Newsboy cap, a shy smile emerges, causing his deep-set eyes to crinkle at the edges. They are the brown of polished oak, and they twinkle like the only two stars giving light to an otherwise cool, dark night. The hat reveals an almost bald head. I'm pretty sure I never told Cheryl that I have a thing for bald men. I see a narrow, straight nose, rosy, lush lips, broad shoulders, and a head that would be a shame to cover up with hair. My suspicion was wrong. Oh my gosh, this guy is adorable.

We decide that he will ride with me. That way I can head home after dinner and he can ride back with Chipper and Cheryl. As I drive, we chat. He's fidgeting with his watch and I'm gripping the steering wheel like it's a raft in the rapids. I ease up on my grip and try to pay attention to our banter. I really don't know what he is saying, because his accent is strong. But damn, is he cute!

We nibble on sushi and make small talk for the next hour and a half. He continues to nervously fidget with his watch between bites. Even though I have a very hard time understanding him, I feel something from his aura that I'm drawn to. I sense a gentle strength, humble yet confident. He has an easy-going energy, but there is something creative and mysterious deep inside him.

Over the next few months, not a day goes by that we don't talk or at least text. We go on dates. I don't want the girls to know, so when I can manage care for Caroline, and when Mike doesn't have his seven-year-old son Konrad, he drives to my office to pick me up and we go out.

I have convinced myself that I could never invite a man into a lifetime of caring for Caroline. I rationalize that there will never be one forever man for me. We would have little hope for spontaneity, freedom, or the glory of the empty nest days.

And yet, after three dates, I know this isn't casual. Or is it that I can't do casual? My daydreams—or shall I call them my cardio dreams—they are about love. I dream of loving a man who is confident, strong yet gentle, affectionate, creative, and fun. Definitely fun. I imagine a man who wants me, in all the ways a lover desires a partner. Never in these cardio dreams do I dream of many men. It's one man.

The thing about dating from my office, rather than my home, is that it's not like I can say, "Would you like to come inside?" I mean, would we just sit there at my conference table in two Office Depot chairs, playing Jenga with the sleeves of staples? But on the fourth date, I do have a thought.

"Would you like to come inside and see my office?" I ask Mike as we pull into the parking lot. I still can't understand a lot of what he says, but I clearly hear, "Sure!"

I show him my office, the accountant's office, the reception area, the conference area, the bathroom, and the little kitchen. That's all there is to it. But it's mine, and I'm proud of it. He remarks on each space and asks some questions about workflow that have never crossed my mind. I'm guessing that's an engineering thing. Or a German thing. It's sure not a Tara thing.

When we get to the door to leave, he turns back to face me and asks, "Do you know what I like best in here?"

I start to answer, but I'm stopped as two strong arms wrap around me and the softest, most sensuous kiss envelops me. It tastes like sunrise. His breath, the heat, the softness of those lips—I don't want it to end. But when it does, I surprise myself. I pull back just enough to see the smile on this man's face, and those twinkling eyes. I say, "There is something I have been wanting to do since I met you."

"And what is that?" Mike asks.

I take hold of his face and gently pull it down toward me. I rise up to my toes and remember that I choose joy. Ever so softly, I kiss the crinkle at the outside corner of Mike's eye. He smiles, the crinkles dance, and my heart beats a little melody made for skipping through town on a spring morning.

CHAPTER 23
DEATH TO NICOTINE

It's been more than a year since that first date with Mike. My life now has a source of joy that is not tethered to duty or trauma. I've learned that if I'm going to keep fighting for Caroline and showing up for her with patience and intention, I also need time away. Away from the house, my phone, my work. . . and her. Needing time away from Caroline is hard to accept. It's harder to write, but it is the truth.

I used to intuit that I didn't deserve anything that resembled happiness unless it was in pursuit of fighting for or delivering happiness to one of my children. But now I see that freedom and joy are not to be earned. They are right there within my grasp, right between the work and the heartache. Perhaps I unknowingly learned this as a child who preferred to jump off the high dive. My aspiring ballerina brain was called to the split-second opportunity between springing off the board and splashing into the water. It's why I used to leap with a *grand jeté* into the air, holding freedom for as long as gravity would allow.

It's just before 3 p.m. as I drive back from working in my territory. I have already changed into my leggings and sweatshirt in the RaceTrac bathroom. I take pride in how I have mastered the art of never letting my bare feet or an article of clothing touch the floor as I change in a public restroom. I'm on my game today. I have an hour to spend at Oconee Veteran's Park, then back at my office from 4:00 until 5:25. I can be home just in time for Michelle to leave promptly at 5:30. I strap on my pink mini iPod, tuck my key in my sports bra, and I'm off. I'm feeling the Dixie Chicks[2] today. Like a normal human, I walk through the front of this park that is made up of walkways, baseball fields, and a concession stand. I'm not normal, though. I have a secret, and it's in the back of this park. I smile as Natalie Maines sings that she's ready to run because she wants to be free.

That's right. For the next hour, I am free. Free to unleash. Free to celebrate. I'm now at the back of the park, the place where normal people think it ends. But it doesn't. I stare out at mounds of red Georgia clay. It's been graded or something like that. But it just sits here, its motionless hills and valleys calling me. There is only one tiny sign that says, "Do not enter." But hell, anyone could miss that sign, right? These hills were meant to be climbed and danced upon. And that is exactly what I do. I greet the hills with pirouettes and *grand jetés*. My body is trying to celebrate a freedom and love that it can't contain. And so, I skip, leap, twirl, and sing through the dirt mounds. I feel like a fairy princess who just discovered her wings.

---

[2] Today known as The Chicks

Singing and driving my way back to the office, I whip the Expedition into my parking space and jump out of the seat with a *zip-a-dee-doo-dah* kind of step.

I'm in love. I tried to warn Mike, to push him away from my future, but he wouldn't hear of it. His love makes my worst days easier to survive. And it makes my best days play out in colors more vibrant than I have yet to see.

Some days this love propels me like I'm Tinker Bell on a mission. But on the days that are tarnished with sadness, Mike's love feels like a safety cushion. Only weeks ago, he helped me take Caroline to the hospital because a seizure had dislocated her shoulder. I had gripped his hand and covered my mouth with his shoulder as the young doctor tried once, then twice, and on the third try, finally snapped Caroline's shoulder back into place. When we finally got her resting in bed that night, I collapsed onto the cold tile of my kitchen floor. And he didn't run. He just let me feel. He held me close. And then he held me up. Even when he's working on another continent, I feel him holding me up, and at the same time setting me free.

I'm walking into my office, still all sweaty and slightly breathless. Everyone is gone for the day except Brad, my sales associate. He is stuffing his laptop into his backpack when he looks up and smiles his magical smile.

"Tara Belle!" you must have been out running like Phoebe again. "You look so, um, happy."

He is referring to how I shared with him that ever since Billy moved out, my cardio dreams were no longer unattainable fairy tales. They transformed into an exploding kind of energy, *the energy of hope*. And this made me want to dance. So I would go out and not really run, but leap and twirl about like I did today. It reminded me of Phoebe from the episode of *Friends* where she embarrassed Rachel by showing her how to run and dispel boredom. She flailed about, spastically flinging her limbs as she traveled through Central Park, showing Rachel what fun and freedom look like.

"You know it, baby," I say to Brad with a grin.

"Let's go to the mall," he says, as he slings his backpack over his shoulder.

"What?" I ask. "I have ninety, well now really eighty minutes to get through these orders and reload before tomorrow. And I can't make it out to the mall and back in time to let Michelle leave."

"I thought you were Miss Run-like-Phoebe, spontaneous Tara today. Come on. I'll call Michelle from the car and ask her to stay late. Let's go. I'm driving."

"Brad, what the hell is at the mall?" I giggle. "You know I'm a snob, right? I don't shop in that shithole."

He laughs, "Well today you're going to walk among us commoners. Let's go. You'll see."

Brad is speed-walking through Macy's, past Victoria's Secret, Old Navy, the Footlocker, and the Great American Cookie Company. He finally slows down. "There it is." He points to a kiosk with two guys standing in front of it.

"Hey, man," Brad says to the tallest one. "This is my boss. She needs to quit smoking. Show her the eCig!"

He is right. I do want to stop smoking. I feel it killing me. It fucks up my running-like-Phoebe; I am tired of how it controls me. And oddly, for the first time, I actually think I could do it. I'm a little afraid of outgrowing all my clothes, because the last time I quit smoking, I gained 10 pounds in about six weeks. I guess that could have been because I replaced my cigarettes with Brown Sugar Cinnamon Pop-Tarts.

One hundred and fifty dollars later, I am walking out of the mall with my new eCig. Brad and I laugh all the way to the parking lot. When we get in his truck, I pull it out of the box and glance over at him.

"Go ahead!" he urges. "The guy said you can smoke it indoors. It evaporates and doesn't leave an odor. Let's see it!"

I inspect the slender silver tube that is slightly heavier and longer than a Marlboro Light. I raise it up to my lips and try to inhale. But my lips won't let me. Neither of us can stop laughing. Brad drives and I keep trying, but the laughter is winning.

Finally, I say, "Okay, this is serious shit. Say something serious. I will focus and then I will quick-like-a-fox suck on this baby." And we crack up again. I catch my breath, but then I have to put the magic eCig down, to cover my face and look away from a still-laughing Brad. "Maybe you should slap me. I will cry, then want a cigarette and I can just suck on this thing."

"I'm not slapping my boss. Just get a hold of yourself, Tara Belle. Go."

And with that, I turn my head toward my window, put the cylinder to my lips and inhale. The end of it lights up like the blue light on a police car, and so, of course, my exhale is in the form of more laughter.

I block the peripheral view of Brad with my left hand, bite into my cheeks, and then say, "Shut up. Stop laughing. I think this could work. I like it! Just drive, asshole."

And that day was the beginning of the end of my love affair with Marlboro Lights. It took time, but one day I smoked my last real cigarette and didn't buy another pack. For several more weeks, I just stuck to the eCig until one evening when I was sitting on my bed. Everyone was asleep. Rather than going out on the porch, I went into my bedroom, took the sleek cylinder off its charger, sat down on my bed, and inhaled. It crackled and chugged. No blue light. No vapor entered my lungs. I tapped and tightened it. The front of it was fried. Literally. And that's when I realized I was done. The eCig had died.

"Better you than me, baby," I said to the lifeless old friend. I threw it in the bathroom trash can, got into my bed, and picked up my cell phone to text Billy:

"I want to run the Peachtree Road Race with you next year. Can you sign me up, too?"

CHAPTER 24
BENZO-MANIA

The schools are closed for Good Friday, so I work at my office all morning and then sneak away for a run and to hang out at Mike's house. It's amazing how the lungs can improve when you don't fill them with smoke, tar, and nicotine. I have just returned from running with Mike's dog, a huge black Labradoodle named Wolfie. I didn't know dogs could be so different from Bruiser, or all the other Boxers I grew up with. Boxers are spastic. Their excitement for the pleasures of life takes over their bodies as if they were given a triple espresso and then released from jail. Wolfie is no Boxer. I run for miles with him, and he stays right beside me. I feel like I'm such a hip chick when I'm out running with him. Me, my smoke-free lungs, and this cool-ass dog whose shiny, black coat dances in tandem with his gait.

Wolfie and I return to find Mike in his garage, which is also a workshop. He's wearing safety glasses and overalls, and he's covered in sawdust. When he sees me, he pulls off the goggles and walks toward me. His dusty hands grab my sweaty face and he kisses me as if I've been gone for a week. I melt into this kiss and realize, I found him—the imaginary man from my cardio dreams. He is right here, holding my face, kissing my lips. He tastes a little like Nutella. I had never tasted Nutella until I met Mike. I knew my life was missing more than love.

I pull away, "Did you eat Nutella on Harvest Grain bread without me?"

We turn to walk into the house with Wolfie, and Mike replies, "Nein! Nein, Frau Heaton, Nein," as he smacks me on the ass. I fill Wolfie's water bowl and chug a glass myself while Mike slices the Harvest Grain bread.

"I think I need to get home," I say, licking Nutella from a knuckle. "I need to spend some time with Holly. I'm worried about her. Every freaking time she tries to talk to me, we are interrupted by Caroline. Every little noise or movement I hear or even sense, I jump and race to see if Caroline is okay. It's so messed up. I mean, think about it, Mike. Holly was the baby of the family. She's lost that. She needs her mom to let her be the baby."

"But she's not a baby," Mike says. "She will be okay. She's smart, she's—"

"No. It's not okay. You don't see what I see when I look into her eyes. I see anger and a sadness that rips into me. It's a lonely look, with a lot of life experience for a 15-year-old girl. She may appear okay, because she's loud and she always comes in hot and shiny. Plus, she makes excellent grades and she's involved in sports and clubs and shit. My God, of course she's loud. She's trying to be heard. She's trying to remind me that she has needs, too. I think on the inside, she's actually screaming, 'Hell-O! I hurt, too, you know.'"

I try to continue, but Mike simply pulls me into him. "Oh, my Sunshine," he says as he removes my ball cap and strokes my head. "She will be okay. Her mom is Tara Heaton."

And then Tara Heaton does something she thought she forgot how to do. She weeps. It's not the urge of sobbing in horror at Caroline's pain. It's more peaceful, a satisfying release. I try to pull away, to be strong. To be Tara Heaton. But Mike firmly holds me there, and I give in. I cry into his chest as if I'm the little girl Holly needs to be.

I finally pull back, wipe my face with a paper towel, put my cap back on and say, "I'm telling you, this little girl needs her mom."

I kiss Mike, kiss Wolfie, and with a big, teary grin, kiss Mike again.

With that he says, "Gross. Get out of here, woman."

I'm driving down Barnett Shoals Road toward home, completely devoted to a lightning-fast shower and sneaking only Holly out of the house. *We are going to treasure some life minutes today, my baby girl.*

As I think this, my phone rings. It's Holly! I flip it open and answer, "Hi Honey. I'm on my way home. Be ready to—"

"Mom!" she screams. "Mom! Get home. Caroline! She's freaking out! What is wrong with her?"

My nervous system shifts into speed-mode.

"I'm coming, Honey. I'm so sorry. Almost there. Tell Michelle I'm five minutes out."

"Just hurry up!" She ends the call.

I slam the Expedition into park in the driveway and run through the garage and into the kitchen.

Caroline is sitting on the couch and Michelle is standing over her, looking pale and petrified.

From a swollen face, Caroline is screaming at Michelle, "No! No! I hate you. I hate everyone!" And she starts slapping her thighs. Then she begins ripping at her hair. "I'm stupid. See? I used to be smart, but now I'm stupid. My brain is stupid. I just want to go away!"

As I beg Caroline to stop, to calm down, I feel Holly behind me. She steps in front of me and buries her sweet, rosy face in my boney chest. Poor baby. In this moment, I wish I was plumper, softer, a kinder place for a little girl to be cradled. For only an instant, I hold her head and stroke her hair as she whimpers.

I pull away from Holly to control Caroline. I grab her hands so she will stop hurting herself.

"Michelle, I'm going to take Caroline to the hospital and I'm not leaving it until someone helps us. She is not safe. I will figure this out, I promise. Could you please stay with Holly? Do anything to take her mind off this. Please. Give her a reason to smile. Here's my credit card. Do whatever y'all want."

Right as we pull out of the subdivision, Caroline unbuckles her seatbelt and tries to climb out the window. I reach for her shirt, but it just stretches as if she can climb out of it, too. I grab again. I grab her hair. I'm steering with my left hand, pulling on my daughter by her hair and now we are both screaming. I order her to calm down as I stop the car in the middle of the street. I pull again, just enough to get the window up. She screams back in response to the pain of my yanking her thinning hair. I feel like a monster. Who grabs their child by the hair? She needs help. How do I get her safely to that help?

"I hate you. Let me out! Let me out!"

With both hands, she slaps at her face. She pulls her hair again and then yanks her thin, gold-hoop earrings until one comes loose. She tries to fling it out the window, but I have locked it, so her hand slams into the glass and she screams again.

"Caroline. Please listen to me. I'm going to get you help. Honey, you have too much medication in your little body. It's making you feel this way. You will feel better soon, I promise. Please, please try to stay calm. I'm going to find someone to help you."

She stops clawing at herself and I drive on. She digs her fingers into her jeans on either side of her thighs and starts rocking her torso, forward toward the windshield and then slamming back into the car's headrest.

These fucking drugs! I'm enraged with a heat that burns my chest. I feel like a fool. Besides countless neurologists, we have seen a dietician, a naturopath, a functional medicine expert, and a homeopath. We've been to a chiropractor, an acupuncturist, and a hyperbaric chamber clinic. And let us not forget the insane mom who traveled across the country and lived in a Marriott for three weeks for the holy grail—biofeedback. All these quirky Zen masters have one united message: Synthetic drugs are an antagonist to healing.

"Caroline! please," I half-yell, half-beg. "Listen to me! Remember, I promised. I promised you that I am your warrior for life. I'm fighting for you every day. I will keep searching, keep driving, flying, cooking, spending. Whatever it takes! Just try to be patient and trust that I will never, ever give up."

As I pace the floor of the tiny ER room, I feel the urge to put my hands over my ears like a kindergartner. I'm enduring the sound that I hate most on earth, the beeping and chirping of monitors. I want action. Someone, somewhere on this earth must be able to help my daughter.

Finally, a baby-faced, fit-looking doctor arrives. He looks at me and I imagine he sees a crazy woman who needs a Xanax or a fat joint. My thoughts are twisted like a broken Slinky. I cannot tell Caroline's story even one more time.

All I can do is beg, "Please, please help her. She is not safe. She needs to be admitted or something. She is suicidal. She screams. She slaps herself. And for God's sake, please do not give her any more drugs. I think drugs are the problem. She's so drugged up and addicted to benzodiazepines that she is not herself anymore. Do something. Anything. Just please don't send us home. I can't. I can't take her back home."

"Mrs. Heaton," he starts. I suck in all the air I can and hold it there. "I know this is difficult. I can't imagine what you all have been through. But we can't admit her here for psychiatric care. What I'm going to do is refer you to a psychiatrist. The office is closed, but I sent them a note. Call them on Monday if you don't hear from them by about

10 a.m. They will schedule an appointment and work with you to manage Patricia's medication."

"My name is Caroline," Caroline corrects. She remains stiff, arms crossed, staring at the wall in front of her. "Patricia Caroline Heaton. People call me Caroline. Patricia is my Memaw's name. But people call her Pat. I'm Caroline."

Without acknowledging the interruption, little Doogie Houser continues, "That is all we can do, Mrs. Heaton. This is the ER. And from our observation, Patricia, ah, Caroline is not a danger to herself or others."

"Let's go Caroline," I say as I reach over and peel the tape that is holding the I.V. in place.

"Mrs. Heaton, the nurse will do that," says Doogie.

"Riiight," I sneer. "I'm going to do what I always do—do it myself." I grab a tissue that I assume is sterile, place it across Caroline's forearm, and swiftly pull the needle out of her arm.

"Let's go, Patricia Caroline Heaton. We are out of here. These people won't help you, so I will."

Now I'm in warpath mode. As I drive home, I look over at Caroline, who is out of mania and in a trance. Across my tongue and into my throat, I taste the salty acid of determination. Buildings become sparse and the sunset turns the sky the colors of raspberries, tangerines, and lemons. The view is as if we are on an exquisite island. I choose to see it as a sign of affirmation.

I call my little brother Jeff. He doesn't answer, so I leave a voice mail, "I'm ready. We are ready. Let's do it. Let's put Caroline on the wheatgrass diet. Call me."

I end the call and look at Caroline. "Baby, we are going to Hawaii!"

CHAPTER 25
COUNTING CHANGE

The spring of 2010 is managed with a new therapist, more diet restrictions, and of course, more medication. Gone are Caroline's outbursts and erratic behavior. Also gone is any semblance of my first daughter. *This is temporary*, I assure myself. *She is hibernating behind all these drugs. We will endure this until we can go to Hawaii.*

Billy and I are sitting in the last IEP (Individualized Education Plan) meeting of Caroline's senior year. I feel outnumbered at this giant conference table crowded by the principal, guidance counselor, teachers, a paraprofessional, some people from the district office, and the face I prefer to focus on, Miss Faye, the angel of a school nurse. Thankfully, this is Billy's area of expertise. He is an elementary school principal now himself. He knows Caroline's rights. Plus, he can kick me under the table when I start to explode with one of my signature untamed rants. These meetings are micro-presentations delivered with what translate to me as caution and pity. It feels like feigned compassion from some, and true empathy from others.

They are all talking about Caroline's lack of progress, her decline in memory, her impaired cognitive function, and her inappropriate behavior. They show tests, charts, and graphs to validate the fact that our beautiful 18-year-old daughter's brain is slowly deteriorating. And then, like sugary applesauce to disguise a pill, they say how much they love her. I feel patronized as they tout her ability to count the change from the school store.

Mr. Meeks, one of the district people, pastes a smile on his face and speaks in a perfunctory cadence, "She will walk in the graduation ceremony with her friends. She will be presented with a special education diploma."

This is basically a piece of cardstock that says, *I showed up for school the required number of days because my parents got me on the short bus. I sat in my grandpa chair, counting my coins like a good girl. I am rewarded with this worthless piece of paper that leads to nowhere.*

While I let Billy speak the maddening acronym-speak of education, I retreat to envisioning my trusty bucket filled with vases, sitting at the top of our driveway. As the meeting drones on, I focus on the images of big, heavy crystal vases. I scoop one up, plant myself as if I'm up to bat, twist as far as my obliques will allow, and then hurl the vase into the brick wall of our home. I repeat this action in my head again and again. The sound of the smashing glass inside my head drowns out the stoic, reporting voices of all the contributing officials.

When the meeting convenes, I leave all my belongings at my seat and walk straight to Miss Faye. I hug her and whisper, "You have been Caroline's savior. And mine. I will never find the words to thank you." I pull back from the hug and return to collect my purse and the massive stacks of papers we have been gifted. I'm mad. Not at the people gathered at this table. Well kind of, but I know it's irrational. They don't know I'm not really a mom of a special needs child. Caroline tested into the gifted class in fourth grade.

I fold up the stack of papers that prove I am, in fact, a mother of a special needs child. All these education professionals have made my daughter a priority today, yet all I can utter is "thank you."

Feeling hot and queasy, I bolt toward the door. I hear Billy talking to his colleagues, but I keep walking, faster and faster until I am free from those halls and outside in the parking lot. In fairness, I'm not sure what I wanted from them. I reject pity, yet my anger gurgles, looking for an opening to unleash its fury. It's in these warrior-mode moments that I fear letting go of this anger because I fear I will let go of my fight. Somehow, I have fused anger and the fighting spirit.

I'm waiting at my car, trying to let the fresh air ventilate my thoughts, when I see Billy walking toward me.

"Well, I guess those middle school mean girls who predicted Caroline would be in special ed were right all along," Billy says with a grimace. He hugs me. He pulls back and makes that familiar fight-back-tears Billy sound, "Aacchh!" And then he says, "Want to go get a beer?"

I look at my watch. It's still two hours until Michelle leaves. I smile and with an exhale say, "Yes."

"Loco's?"

"See you there."

During the short drive, I'm able to release some of the anger, leaving the glass vases in the high school parking lot. I accept the reality that pain is bound to me, and as I do, I make room for gratitude. The shared pain that only Billy and I can grasp is the source of a rare and precious connection. Our relationship is deeper than ever because of what we have endured. But it's also a symbol of freedom, because of what we are no longer denying. It's as if a part of us has been sleeping, like a black bear preparing for spring. I will continue the journey toward a better life for Caroline, but it cannot be my only dimension. I want Wilson and Holly to see me as a reminder that they are the orchestrators of their own lives. I want them to know that heartache does not disqualify them from living the life that is now.

I click on my new Bluetooth thingamajig and call to check in with the kids. Holly picks up and I tell her I am meeting her dad for an hour before coming home.

She tells me everything is okay there, but wants to know, "Why are you meeting up with dad? Are y'all getting back together?"

My heart skips a beat as I prepare to wipe away what I assume is a flicker of hope. "Oh, Honey, no. Your dad and I have a very special friendship, but that is all that it is. A friendship."

But I misread Holly's sentiment. I didn't wipe away a flicker of hope, I wiped away a moment of worry.

Holly jumps in with, "Okay, good. Everyone is so much happier now."

CHAPTER 26

THE 3 LEGGED COWBOY

Billy and I are settling into a spacious booth at Loco's. I see one of our neighbors a few booths back and imagine she wonders what this divorced couple is doing out for a beer together on a Thursday afternoon. I decide not to care.

We raise our glasses and with my spirit of freedom, I say a tad too loudly, "To love. Cheers."

We clink, sip, and then Billy says with a smile, "How's your boyfriend?"

"So good," I smile back. "How is yours?"

"Tara," Billy starts. "I think I love Channing. He is a fine person and he makes me happy. And he is so open to being more invested in Caroline's life. I think we are going to move in together. The plan is to have a house in Gwinnett County by the time my lease is up."

I have a lot of questions, most of which revolve around our kids.

"I'm really happy for you." I genuinely am. "I'm also obviously wondering about the kids. How do you plan to tell our kids that their dad is gay and has a new life partner? I mean, it's time, right?"

He has clearly given this some thought. "I'm not ready to do that." He plans to tell the kids that Channing is a roommate because he wants a nice home again and the way to do that financially right now is with a roommate. Plus, Bruiser will have a yard again and his children will have a more spacious place to visit.

I sip my beer and imagine this coming into reality. Caroline will not question it. Holly may suspect that her dad and Channing are more than roommates. And Wilson, he will know. I flash back to the night when I lied to Wilson, the night we both pretended. When his dad moves in with a guy who is afraid of bugs and looks like he was made over by the *Queer Eye*'s Tan France, Wilson will know for sure.

Billy excuses himself to take a phone call and I think back to the night I met Channing. Billy wanted me to experience the world he was learning to embrace, to meet some new friends and especially the man he had dated a few times. I didn't hesitate to accept this invitation. I even asked myself why I wasn't opposed or mad or jealous or something that qualifies as a bitter emotion. With courageous honesty, my reaction became clear: Billy's happiness assuaged my guilt about asking him to move out. I had dreamed of true love for years before Billy stopped denying his nature.

My love for Billy was no longer romantic or sexual, and I yearned for romance, intimacy, and a life that explored my sexual being. And so, if I could see that Billy was happy, had friends and community, then I could be released of any guilt. Plus, I was damn curious about this gay, country western, two-step dance club. I mean, who would turn down a chance to dance to "The Watermelon Crawl" with a collective of queens?

That night, I met Billy in the parking lot of the 3 Legged Cowboy. My pulse elevated and my chest tightened with nervous excitement.

With his arm around my shoulder, Billy guided me into his new world. It was a crowded sea of men with a variety of styles. Many looked like your average beer-guzzling, college football fans, wearing polo shirts that stretched over proud bellies and tucked into Old Navy jeans. There were men dressed in cowboy hats, plaid shirts, and tight-fitting Wranglers adorned with bedazzled belt buckles. And there were men strutting about in short skirts, tank tops, and cowboy boots that clicked and stomped to the beat. I saw no drag queens, but I did see a bold, carefree dancing queen in a solid gold sequined hat, turquoise boots with spurs, and a pair of chaps with only a G-string underneath.

Shine on brother, I thought. *You do have a flawless ass.*

But what put an irrepressible smile on my face at the 3 Legged Cowboy was not the attire; it was the dancing. I was mesmerized. Every time the DJ changed the song, the couples gracefully changed their steps and continued with a fresh version of the two-step, all moving to the same easy, upbeat rhythm. I tried to speak, but I was smitten by this joyful playground for men. They gathered there to be themselves, to celebrate freedom without judgment.

I knew that each of these men must have a story that included fear and probably ridicule, shame, and seasons of depression. But one thing was for sure, they had a story that was woven with courage and an intense appreciation for love.

In that moment, I thought, *perhaps we don't choose joy in spite of whatever trauma or grief we have endured.* Rather, it's the magnitude of that suffering that determines the depth of our desire to unapologetically rejoice.

I was caught up in the contagious vibe of the dance bar when Billy tapped my shoulder and introduced me to Channing. It was so loud, I couldn't do more than offer a generic greeting. It could have gotten awkward, but before that could transpire, Billy yelled that he would be back. I heard Sara Evans launch into the first chorus of "Suds in the Bucket."

I watched in astonishment as Channing led my ex-husband around the dance floor. It felt awkward, but I didn't want it to. While this sight was novel to me, Billy was finally embracing how nature had perfectly intended him to be. He was free.

Now here at Loco's, I snap out of the memory as Billy returns to our little booth. Before he can sit back down, I slide out of my seat and kiss his cheek. He doesn't question this randomness. For more than 20 years, he has experienced how I don't resist my urges to express affection. Now it's his turn.

We sit down and I tell him I have two things to discuss. The first is Caroline and her piteous quality of life. He leans in as I share my reasons for why we should plan to take Caroline to see my brother, who lives in Hawaii on his wheatgrass farm.

We recount the past five years. I pull out my list of the drugs we have tried: Dilantin, Klonopin, Felbamate, Vimpat, Lyrica, Phenobarbital, Tegretol, Depakote, Fycompa, Lamictal, Trileptal, Keppra, Gabapentin, Topamax, and Zonegran. I take a breath and then summarize the traditional attempts at seizure control. We started at Emory of Atlanta. We went to Birmingham, Alabama. Then we tried the pediatric epileptologist in Augusta, Georgia. There we had the Vagus nerve stimulator surgery. We have spent two weeks in two different hospitals where they backed off Caroline's drugs until she hit violent seizures that they could monitor. Both times they confirmed that she is not a candidate for a brain dissection, because her seizure origins are multi-focal.

As we lost hope in drugs and procedures, we traveled to Johns Hopkins in Baltimore for the Ketogenic diet. I became a master at frying chicken, coated in mayo, rolled in pork skins. From there we got creative. We flew out to California and spent most of our savings embracing biofeedback.

When that failed, a functional medicine expert put her on an all-natural, sugar-free, zero-processed diet. We went to an acupuncturist, a homeopath, a chiropractor, and we even checked out a hyperbaric chamber.

And today, what do we have to show for it? As I push away my warm beer, I say, "Billy. Caroline is an addict.

Every time her seizures start to cluster, we give her Ativan. As you know, she needs more and more of it to stop the seizures. There is no denying, her seizures have, possibly irreparably, damaged her brain. Based on all I have read, her behavior is classic benzodiazepine addiction. That's what we have allowed these doctors to create. Our poor baby is a drug addict who doesn't understand what her body is craving. We are out of options. And Billy, you know me. I won't sit back and watch this nightmare play out. I have to fight it."

The always-loyal Billy asks about the details. He trusts my research and my brother, but wants to know the risks.

"Here is how I see it, Billy. We just got back from a beach trip, a place Caroline used to love. She spent every evening in a giant purple stroller made for quadriplegics. She complained, she yelled, she argued, she shrieked at her inability to understand. And we only got breaks from this when she would have a seizure and then sleep either on the beach or in the stroller for a while. The trip was sheer misery—for all of us."

I continue, "We returned from that trip and went straight back to the doctor. And as you know, now she is even more sedated. She exists in an emotionless cloud that seems vacant from the inside. So what exactly are we risking? A way of life that we don't want to downgrade?" I force a laugh at the irony and take a swig of the lukewarm ale. "What are we risking? Nothing. Her quality of life is at zero. That's how I see it."

Billy doesn't hesitate. "Let's do it. I agree. And so, when?"

I explain that I can't go until the Christmas holiday

because for one, the schools are out and I won't have to miss so much work. But also, because Wilson will be home from college and I want to take him with us.

"Why? He will miss Christmas, too? It will just be Holly and me?"

I tell Billy that I need him to be with Holly, but I simply can't imagine doing this alone. I will need little breaks. To breathe, to compose myself. Plus, Wilson is the only person who can still put a smile on Caroline's face. She gives her very best when he is around. And it's no wonder. He is still, to this day, her fierce protector and patient confidant. I need him. And I think so will Caroline."

Billy agrees and then I have one more piece of news.

"And now on to something that I hope will delight you," I say.

"I could use some delight," he confirms.

"Where is the place on earth you want to see? More than any city in the world, where do you want to go?"

He laughs and says, "You already know. London. Before I die, I will see London. I will stand before Windsor Castle and yell, 'Hail to the queen!'"

I start to laugh. "I told Mike about your obsession with Princess Diana and the entire royal family. He just shook his head at me and said, 'Yet still, you had no clue your husband was gay.'"

Billy chuckles and I continue, "The news is that I have won a trip to London with my company."

"Oh wow, I'm happy for you. That's amazing," he says. He starts to discuss the historical places I might visit.

"Billy, you're not getting the point. It took three years for my business to take off. It was grueling. It was trips, long nights, and early mornings. And as it grew, the demand for me to be gone increased. And you, you were always there, never once complained. I could never have grown this business without you and I would not have won a fancy trip to London. You are going with me. You are going to London, Mr. Heaton."

Billy tried to resist, asking about Mike, why I'm not taking him, and how he might feel.

But I wasn't taking no for an answer. "It's all settled, assuming your parents can keep the girls. Actually, what I would like to do is fly from London to meet Mike in Germany and spend a few days with his family. I'll go from London with my ex-husband to Bavaria with my boyfriend." I grin.

Billy looks like he's starting to believe me.

"Screw what's typical, Billy. This is us. This is the beautiful new family we are building. I have even inquired about twin beds! I'm taking you, my best friend, the 3 Legged Cowboy's dancing queen, to London!"

CHAPTER 27
TWO MEN AND A TRIP

While flying across the English Channel on the way to Munich, I think back over the past five days in London. Gratifying. That is how I would describe seeing Billy in a constant state of awe as we explored London together. The next best part was the day we split up and I went shoe shopping on Oxford Street. That felt indulgent, frivolous, and fabulous. And thankfully so, because the food was anything but fabulous. It mostly tasted like fried dishtowel, hold the spice, double the mayo. Cheerio, Brits!

Now I'm headed for the land of sunflowers and biergartens.

I peer out my plane window into the abyss of clouds. Something about being alone on an airplane makes me feel free. Ironically, I'm not free; I'm trapped by the massive man sleeping beside me, with access to earth controlled by the pilots. Freedom in this moment is internal—I am unable to fill any of the obligations of life. I can't call doctors, therapists, teachers, or rehab facilities. I can't work out, do my job, or obsessively research intractable epilepsy.

I can only savor my thoughts and record them if I desire. My mind is free because, in this moment, there is not one single thing I could or should be doing.

Staring out at the clouds, I try to resolve some conflict. Deep in my belly, joy and gratitude are dancing. But a touch of guilt and shame prickle my mind. I want affirmation that I am allowed to embrace delight. But the imaginary *Good Woman Playbook* demons deny me the right to feel happy. They wag a finger in my face, telling me I am restricted from joy because the three young humans at the center of my world have needs. They declare all allowances of happiness will be granted to those who have done a better job at perfecting their lives.

Is goodness defined by our capacity for suffering, with no reprieve, no permission to just let heartache hibernate? These nagging shame demons tell me, *you are not permitted to smile broadly, to laugh with your head thrown back, to orgasm, or to free your spirit to dance across these clouds.*

With endless stamina, the clouds perform a meditative dance that is sensual and proud. From the giant cloud families, fluffy portions partially break away, flutter, and grow. These great manatees of the sky stretch and glide into freedom while remaining connected to their home.

I settle my chin in my hand and let the clouds speak. Never could I disconnect from my family, my home. As mothers, our children are rooted in all that we do. We owe them only one thing—to be a person who lives in accordance with her values. Our children should see that their mom is a woman who can still stand tall, a woman who chooses to embrace life's challenges *and* life's offerings with all her might. If we can't free ourselves to do this, we are suggesting that to become a parent is to abandon yourself.

I choose not to keep life in restraints until Caroline is cured, Holly is free of anxiety, and Wilson is a sober college graduate. I must drink in this life so that I can keep fighting for what I want to change. I am a woman who loves deeply and fights mercilessly. I cannot be that woman if I let guilt and shame tell me to sit down and hide from the sun. I trust my thoughts are not unique. We must all nourish ourselves with the joy that is sprinkled like wild raspberries along our path toward home.

As I walk down the jet bridge into the Munich airport, I realize I only know three German words: *hallo, sonnenschein*, and *flittchen*. I have no need to say, "Hello, you sunshiny slut," so basically, I'm helpless.

I follow the confident crowd onto a train. I decide to exit with the masses when I see it: Zoll/Customs. My heart starts to pound as I make it through with my freshly-stamped passport. The thinning crowd guides me to an escalator that descends into a new sea of travelers and greeters. I'm off the belt and into the crowd when I see him and make my way to the twinkling eyes. I feel the urge to kiss the crinkles, but I don't have the chance. Mike gently, firmly puts his palms to my face and pulls my lips to his. He pulls back, searches my eyes, runs his thumb over my irrepressible smile, and then wraps his arms around me. I feel him breathe me in and whisper, "My sunshine."

Go ahead and hibernate, I say to my grief and responsibilities. Just take a back seat, because the next five days are about fortifying my soul. I will meet you back in Georgia and we will get back in the fight.

I hike through sunflower fields, climb majestic mountains, explore castles and bakeries, linger in endless varieties of spectacular flowers, and enjoy a very jolly family that seems to celebrate togetherness with ease and gratitude. Some of Mike's family members speak a little English, but his mom, not at all. Even so, I fall in love with this woman. Her spirit is patient and compassionate. Her voice warms me like a savory stew topped with buttered cornbread. The rest of the family (all younger than this magnificent matriarch), relax and tell stories that spark raucous laughter.

But Mike's mom, she just keeps moving, ensuring every inch of the house is clean, cozy, and filled with fresh flowers, homemade German dishes, warm rolls, and a variety of cakes and pies. Her life had not been an easy one; yet she keeps this kind, generous spirit about her. She gives real hugs that let me understand Mike a little bit better. He's like her, a product of this family. When he is with you, he is fully present, there to enjoy the moment as if he is weaving a keepsake. And like his mom, he loves through actions and affection. He expresses his love with few words, but abundantly through limitless acts of support and intentional touch.

And now, it's just a sweet memory. Mike and I are flying back from Germany together, headed back to reality. I feel the obligation list start to mount. And piled at the top of that list is that feeling again. Guilt. I have to express it to Mike. One more time. He's fumbling with the little swag bag filled with a sleep mask, a wet wipe, two whole Tic Tacs, and a toothbrush made for a baby doll. I gently take the crap-bag out of his hands, forcing him to look at my face.

"Please think long and hard," I say quietly. "Think about your future, your freedom. Caroline will be my responsibility until the day I die. I think I love you too much to let you sign up for that. I'm trying to love you enough to dump you." I smile, but Mike does not smile back.

Mike has a way of saying nothing that invites me to continue.

"You cannot blindly welcome this into your life, your future," I say. "This, this seizure disorder, it's like watching your child slip away as if she has Alzheimer's or something. It's not how life was designed. I'm afraid enduring this will slowly change the Tara you love."

I take a breath.

"Are you done yet?" Mike asks. "This again? It's getting offensive. I love you. Either we are partners or we aren't. I say we are and that means I'm with you. No doubt about it. I have no concerns about growing old and caring for Caro. None. It's my choice. Now shut up about it."

I see Mike's eyes saying *but*. I stare into them as he finds the courage to say it. "If something happens to us because of one of your children, it won't be your daughter . . . it will be your son."

I feel like a concrete sack was just deposited on my chest.

"Tara. Your son has a problem with alcohol. As long as you are his supporter, his co-dependent, he won't face the truth. You keep bailing him out. If you don't let him finally fall, he will never see that he needs to rise up."

I hand the swag bag back to Mike and retrieve my own sleep mask. As I snap it on, I put my head back and try to make space for Mike's words.

After some fitful hours of dozing, I see Mike's eyes open from a pseudo-nap and I decide to change gears. "So," I start. "So. Hawaii. You know I'm serious, right?" He rubs his eyes.

He removes the little neon ear plugs he keeps for walking factories at work and says, "What? Hawaii with your brother, right? Can you tell me again why you think this is a good idea?"

In this airplane, I am aware that we have nothing but time. I take advantage of it as I share my brother's journey. I give Mike the elaborate story of Jeff's history and how many people he has healed with wheatgrass, wheat grain, clay, and well water. He has talked at length with his teacher and mentor about Caroline. This sage has agreed to be on standby all hours of the day as we ween Caroline off her drugs and introduce *health as a form of healing*.[3]

I then try to rationalize what may sound like desperation. "I see it like this. We are out of options from the

---

[3] This diet should not be viewed as healing or medical advice of any kind. The extensive and necessary details are not provided in this book. The wheatgrass, wheat grain, clay, and water regimen should not be considered without research, nor without a doctor's care.

medical community. Trust me when I tell you there is not anything left to uncover that has any empirical evidence of stopping Caroline's seizures. Her quality of life is so low that I think it is simply worth the risk." I take a quick pause. "But I really want to know what you think. I would like to have your support, but I also know that you, above anyone I know, will tell me your honest opinion."

Mike looks at the little screen on the seat in front of him and then turns his body slightly and looks straight at me. "It doesn't matter what I think. You are not looking for my input. I know you. It's already decided. There is no stopping you." And then he smiles and runs his hand through my hair. "But if you want to know what I think, I say go for it. Go to Hawaii, Tara. I hope it brings you home with a happy, drug-free, seizure-free Caro who is ready to get off the couch and back to life."

His hands hold my face, he kisses my lips, and smiles into my eyes. "Now put it out of your head, my woman. It's decided. You are going to Hawaii. I will stay here and invite my forty Eskimo women over to keep me warm while you are gone."

"You freak," I retort. I intertwine my fingers with Mike's, squeeze his hand, and rest my head back against the seat.

CHAPTER 28
A SOLDIER WITH TEARS

The breeze and the peace of the night settle me onto the porch where I try to envision Hawaii. While I've learned not to cling to it like the end-all panacea, I am fueled by it—the energy of hope tied to action.

Imagining us in Hawaii gives me images of beaches, trails, and sunsets. Caroline has loved the beach for as long as I can remember. But our beach trips have changed. I remember the first beach trip after the encephalitis. It wasn't a family beach trip—it was a cheerleading competition on the west coast of Florida. Sure, Holly had to be there, but no way was I going to let Caroline go. Why would I force her to endure watching other girls do something that she so desperately wanted to do again? No way.

But she saw it differently. And so did Casey, the owner of the cheer gym. Casey called and told me that Caroline is still one of them, one of the blue and black United Bulldog cheerleaders. She can be a part of everything except—well, the cheering. Caroline begged to go. I gave in.

When we arrived, Holly went straight to practice with her squad. Caroline and I got settled and then Lauren, one of the coaches, greeted us in the lobby with hugs and took Caroline's hand. I followed behind, wondering why I was allowing this. I was afraid of the lights, the sounds, the total *spasmatic* atmosphere. But mostly I was afraid of it breaking Caroline's heart.

We walked down corridors until we got to the door marked United Bulldogs, Athens, Georgia. Lauren pulled open the door and we stepped into the giant ballroom where all 70 cheerleaders, ages 7 to 17 were lined up, uniforms on, ready to practice. I had to admit, it was good to see all those smiles, even if they were coated in lipstick and Vaseline. Most of them gave a quick, excited wave to Caroline and returned to the ready position. I grabbed Caroline's hand, but she snatched it away.

One of the moms came to hug me and whispered, "Let her stay there. We are right here behind her. Let her sit with the coaches. She's okay."

The coach nodded, put her arm around Caroline, and said, "We've got this, don't we Caroline?"

Caroline looked so happy to be back in this environment. I tried to smile.

Now sitting on the floor with the other cheer moms, I wrapped my arms around myself and stared at 70 royal blue skirts and cropped tops on cheerleaders frozen in anticipation, waiting for the beat of the music. No one moved. I looked directly at Holly, head down, shoulders back, arms stiff, legs locked.

The silence was broken by Miss Casey: "Ready on eight. Five, six, seven, eight!" Seventy curly ponytails popped up and the music blared.

A sea of little athletes thrust their hips from side to side, arms, shoulders, and chests pumping to the beat. In tandem, they dropped to the ground and powered into the air. Fingertips tapped straddled toes. The girls landed together, spun around, and shot their arms strait out like a T. They froze with their backs facing us.

That's when I lost the battle with my tears. Every little cheerleader had a large, white cursive letter C screen-printed in the center of their back. Seventy Cs seared past my eyes and into my heart. I looked over at Miss Casey. She blew me a kiss and mouthed, "We love you," from across the giant, booming room. I glanced at Caroline, Coach Lauren's arm around her, pointing at the uniforms all emblazoned with a C. In that moment I felt a loving energy that I can still manifest to this day.

I have spent a lot of energy seeing only what I dislike in the world of cheerleading. What a loss of life minutes. I missed the commitment, the discipline, the community, and most of all, the love. Even though I had been internally rejecting this culture, there we were, surrounded by seventy families who were cheering us on, as we battled to win the war on seizures.

That memory was five years ago. I try to recount how many times I promised Caroline that she would get better; that I was her warrior, fighting to the death to get her life back. I wasn't lying to her; I still believe it. We just aren't there. Yet.

Fatigue doesn't hit me when I'm in action mode. It hits me when I stop to digest how long I've been on the losing side of this battle. Epilepsy has taken much more than life minutes from Caroline. She has lost her place as a confident, clear-minded girl who loved her friends, swimming, cheerleading, parties, and the beach.

My tears, they taste like the ocean. They remind me that we don't run out of tears, the ocean doesn't dry up; it will always be there when Caroline is ready to love it again. The ocean can be ferocious, and it can be calm, but it keeps moving, flowing with a strength that is eternally replenished because that's how it was created to be. I think back to my nine-year-old self; I feel the flame in my belly, and I know that I too will keep moving, because it's how we are created to be.

I'm ready to bid the porch and the memories goodnight when the kitchen door opens. I quickly reach up and wipe warm tears from my cheeks as Holly walks toward me. The moonlight helps me see that she is crying.

"Holly? What's wrong, Honey? Why are you awake?"

She climbs into the swing beside me, I put my arm around her, and she snuggles close. "The phone rang. It was Wilson. He was yelling at me, but I couldn't understand him. I was going to come get you, but he hung up." My body stiffens and she continues. "But that's not why I'm crying. Then I couldn't go back to sleep."

I feel so desperate to jump off this porch swing and try to reach Wilson. I am tempted to leave Holly and her tears on this porch alone. Wilson needs me. Holly needs me, too.

I grab the chain that holds the swing with my left hand and pull Holly closer with my right.

"What's wrong?" I ask.

"Mom," she begins, and I can hear her voice quiver. "Please don't leave during Christmas. I don't want to be here all by myself. It's . . ." She squeaks out, "It's Christmas!"

Rather than taking my heart out of this moment, I just let it hurt. My jaw clenches and my eyes pierce forward. I feel like a soldier who must leave one child and head off to war to fight for the life of another. And I must remain on this swing, letting one child know her pain matters too, while another child may be in danger.

"Holly, you won't be here by yourself. Your dad will come and stay at the house. He will bring Bruiser. And you will have a wonderful Christmas at Memaw's house."

And then I say three words that should never be used in this order: *I'm sorry, but.*

"I'm sorry but" says we are not really sorry, rather we are telling someone to suck it up, that their feelings aren't valid. And yet, it came right out of the mouth of this soldier.

"I'm sorry, but you understand, my work is in the schools. So I need to leave when school is out. The only other option is to wait until next summer. You see the state that Caroline is in. I can't do that. I will leave a few weeks after your sixteenth birthday. And trust me, you will be very happy after your birthday, because I have a big surprise for you."

I have no idea what this big surprise is, but as of this moment, I know there will be one. That seems to placate

Holly a bit. She smiles through her tears and I ask her to tell me she understands.

We walk into the house and I try not to bolt away in a mad search for my phone. I kiss Holly goodnight and immediately try to reach Wilson. He is no longer in Tifton at ABAC. He wasn't successful there and is now giving college another go at Georgia Southeastern in Statesboro. I call. I text. I call again. And again.

I threaten with texts, because his voicemail is full. No reply. I climb into my bed, make sure my ringer is turned all the way up, and try to sleep, knowing that won't happen. I bet he's asleep, passed out somewhere, unprepared for his classes. I don't count sheep. I count the days until Hawaii, thinking it could be transformative for not just Caroline, but for Wilson, too.

Later that morning, Billy calls. "Last night I went and picked Wilson up from someone's house in Athens. He came stumbling out, all bruised and cut up. I could barely look at him without losing it."

I feel so tired in this moment. Tired of begging Wilson to grow up, to get help, to do anything to get his life on track. Tired of pouring out all my words like I'm the motivational speaker-mom of the universe. So I just talk facts.

"Where is he now, Billy? Does he need a hospital? He needs to get back to school."

Billy explains that Wilson drove some buddies to

Athens for the evening and at around midnight, Jared was elected to drive them all back to Statesboro. He ran Wilson's truck off the road and it rolled down a ravine. They miraculously walked away, the truck is totaled, and he has no transportation.

We think this is it, it's rock bottom for our son, and now he will turn his life around. We stuff away the little boy inside Wilson who is still running, chasing adrenaline to keep from facing his grief. We brainstorm solutions for how he will pass his classes and how he will work without a vehicle. We just stick to coordinating schedules and leave the real needs tightly packed and stuffed down deep. I find solace in the fact that we will be together in Hawaii soon, a trip planned for healing.

CHAPTER 29
ALOHA, UNCLE JEFF

My brother Jeff is a lot like our mom. He takes a curious, enamored interest in everyone he meets. But unlike our mom, he has chosen to create a life free of stress and anxiety. He has two great loves: music and health. He makes a living with music and has devoted his life to the discovery of nature's potential to heal.

My kids light up in the presence of Uncle Jeff. He seems to hydrate their hearts with the way he delights in every detail of their voices, ideas, perspectives, and dreams. And so, even Caroline's spirits are slightly better as we head to Kauai.

During the long, seizure-ridden flights, I remind myself of what I know. For years now, we have been calling the doctor every time Caroline has more than one seizure in a day. The doctors recommend we have her pop the little white pill, Ativan (the brand name for lorazepam). The little white pill stopped working, so they prescribed bigger little white pills. And bigger again.

The Addiction Center publishes that abruptly discontinuing Ativan may cause "severe withdrawal symptoms including seizures, hallucinations, and psychotic reactions.[4]"

Even so, the doctors never hinted to me that they were prescribing the makings of an addict. It was only through my research that I realized why Caroline keeps oscillating between anger and confused lethargy. It's not as simple as depression and anxiety due to loss and trauma. She is seeking that dopamine high that Ativan can provide, yet she's unaware that she is craving the demon that is causing her torment.

We rented a house the size of a New York apartment. In a single room we have a queen bed, a pullout sofa, and a kitchen, plus one door to a tiny bathroom. The low ceilings, dim lighting, and ancient appliances remind me that Hawaii is for getting out, not staying in.

To feel grounded and hopeful about this new treatment, I review the facts in my head. There is clear evidence that organic, ground-grown wheatgrass is nature's fastest-acting healer. It has elastic nutrients that expand to absorb toxins and eating the sprouted wheat aids in sending the toxins out of the body. But wheatgrass can't do this rapidly alone. Clay and spring water alkalize the body and act as a filter by extracting inflammatory pathogens, making room for the growth of healthy cells.

Simply put, AEDs (anti-epileptic drugs) work to lower

---

4 "Ativan Withdrawal and Detox," *Addiction Center*, last modified January 15, 2024, https://www.addictioncenter.com/benzodiazepines/ativan/withdrawal-detox/.

the excitability of nerve cells in the brain. But at the same time, they are toxic and build up in the body, creating a feeding ground for mania and imbalance of the nervous system. So a pure diet of earth, seed, leaf, and water in the form of clay, grain, grass, and water should be able to temper the electrical imbalance in Caroline's brain and reduce her toxic state.

Epilepsy is a nervous system disorder and clay can inhibit the growth of harmful cells in the nervous system specifically. Plus, I personally know a lady who stayed with Jeff and lived this diet because she had pancreatic cancer. The doctors had given her 12 months to live. If this diet could wipe away pancreatic cancer, I have to believe it could eliminate a few misfires in the brain of an 18-year-old girl.

So, with Jeff, his mentor, Caroline's doctor, and a specialist all on standby, I believe we are prepared for the seizures that, unless they cluster, we won't buffer with more Ativan.

In the pit of my gut, I feel like I'm risking my child's life to save her. But again, what life? I have met one too many epileptics who have followed their neurologists' medication protocol for decades. When I think about willingly resigning Caroline's life to an escalating protocol of mind-numbing pharmaceuticals, I know there is no way we could have not come to Hawaii. The doctors have run out of medications to try. The homeopathic alternatives have a success rate of zero.

The only option left is to accept the fate of letting seizures and drugs slowly kill the girl inside the fragile bones, the flawless skin and the face that has come to emanate misery. I know that accepting a more compliant, passive approach to caring for Caroline would also kill the mom with the fighting spirit, leaving only a soulless woman, incapable of empathy or love. So I trusted the embers burning inside me, and here we are.

I don't think Caroline would have agreed to what she is eating for anyone else on earth. But it's Uncle Jeff. Each morning, he shows up with a metal bowl the size of a bass drum. It's filled with a blended concoction of wheatgrass, sprouted wheat, and clay that looks like a greenish-brown poop pudding. At first, Caroline eats it and drinks the muddy clay water without a single complaint. But she soon feels the effects of drugs being evacuated from her body.

The second, third, and fourth days are almost sleepless. Yes, there are seizures, but it's the detoxing that keeps Caroline in a state of mania. With no warning, she catapults out of a deep sleep into a state of mind-altering fear. She throws her body from one side of the bed to the other, and then thrashes into the fetal position and back out again. Intermittently, she begs in a low voice I have never heard before: "Help me. Please. Please help me."

During these first few days, Caroline only takes naps of about 90 minutes, wakes in a state of mania and has seizures. I am in constant contact with our support team and they assure me this will soon pass. Even so, when she starts to actually sleep, it's alarming. The sun wakes me up and I realize I have been sleeping deeply. I cradle Caroline for a moment, and she peacefully groans.

With Wilson asleep on the couch, I scramble to the coffee maker, brew a quick cup, and take it out onto the tiny patch of pavement outside the house. The sun warms me, it smiles at me, reminding me it is a Hawaiian sun, and that I am sitting in one of the most majestic places on earth. I drink in the peace, keep checking on Caroline, and return to this little patch of pavement.

Through the screen door I hear, "Mom? Where are you? Mom?"

I abandon my coffee and race over to the bed. Caroline sits up and looks around the room like a baby deer opening her eyes to discover the forest for the first time. Her speech is slow, as if the effort to speak is tiresome. I remind her that we are in Hawaii to try a special diet with Uncle Jeff. We review the past few days, the plane rides, the long drive. It's not registering. I'm not sure if she doesn't remember or she isn't computing. She looks lost, but she isn't upset. And that look of scalding torment is gone.

With each day, Caroline becomes more at ease, not joyful, but not miserable, either. She is skinny, weak, and wobbly. We want to get her up and out of this dreary hut, out where she can elevate her healing with the beauty and sun that surrounds us. Jeff drives us to a little haven on the coast. We slowly traverse the deep, fine white sand of Kauapea Beach.

Caroline is slow, but she keeps moving. I put down my little tote that holds the untouched emergency Ativan and a jug of clay water. While she waits in a bit of a trance, I spread out our two thin towels. We sit down together and look out at the splashing, teal-blue ocean. I look over at Caroline.

Ever so slightly, she smiles.

Before long, Caroline is asleep again and Wilson is out exploring. Here I am, on a beach in Hawaii, with the energy of hope misting my soul. The clouds tango with the sun as the waves pull the marshmallowy foam farther from our toes. The flow of the ocean soothes me as I mirror Caroline's peaceful breathing and think about the past five days. Sometimes the extreme is the only choice there is. When I imagine living inside the person who didn't choose courage, there is no choice at all.

I roll over onto my front and scoot just close enough to Caroline to feel her breathe. With my chin propped on my palms, I meld my breath with the folding and crashing of the waves.

My meditative trance is interrupted by a graceful, carefree mother and preschool-age daughter. The mother is skimming her toes across the shoreline as she watches her daughter dig in the sand. Look at us. Two moms, here on the beach with our daughters. I wonder if they would like to come over to our hut and have some tea and poop pudding? I study the face that pleasingly stares at her daughter. I want to tell her to hold on tightly, to scoop up that little bundle of fairy tale faith and bask in the ease of this day. But then I see, she already knows. She is right here, right now, playfully savoring her life minutes.

The island of Kauai seems to pulse with a sporadic, aimless melody. Clockless people mosey to work, selling their jewelry or burritos, or not. There is no sales quota, no need to earn a loyal customer. With no urge to conquer or control, they flow with the tempo of the day.

Wilson embraces this vibe completely. It's like his fighting spirit was unleashed to celebrate its very existence. Each day he heads out on a borrowed, single-gear bicycle and stays gone for hours. He returns covered in sand, salt, and enchantment. One particular afternoon, he comes barreling in, letting the screen door slam. His eyes are wide and he's more breathless than usual. I can feel the boom of his heart as his muscles and skin pulse with life. He is telling me that he had gone too far into the current and came close to being swallowed by the sea.

I should be listening more intently, realizing that he should not swim alone. But I'm not really listening to his story; I'm just watching him, inhaling him, and thinking back to the curious, adventure-seeking little boy. I remember his bounding into the house one day when he was about seven, holding a snake. Same breathless energy, same pulsation of skin and muscles. He was fearless, fully invigorated, just like this day in Kauai.

While I understand Wilson's ability to embrace the spirit of Hawaii, it's a challenge for me. Even though Caroline's seizures have stopped, I am nowhere near believing she's not going to crash down at any moment. My shoulders are raised, breath shallow, scalp tight, and I can't take my hands off her. She's gained back some energy, so we go out for short hikes. I'm both encouraged and tormented, because the entire time we're walking, I'm envisioning her catapulting to the dirt, the rocks, the embankment, or the ocean below. She is also very spacey. But what she is not, is angry, which ignites a flickering celebration underneath my heart.

With my hand always in Caroline's, we venture out, explore Kauai. She maintains that graceful, relaxed smile I first saw on the beach. And as each day passes, her eyes become a bit more alive. It's as if she has been sleepwalking for years and is slowly waking up. I can see her again, the girl I have been grieving. I have to trust that in time, she will come out of this trance.

With only a week to go, I call Kathleen to report the miracle of a peaceful Caroline who is drug-free and has not had a seizure in eight days. She listens and asks questions as I prepare to do something that takes me off balance. It's going to take strength, yet it makes me feel weak.

I'm going to ask for help.

I explain to Kathleen that the wheatgrass is working. We need to come home, but it's too soon to move to a raw, organic diet. I force myself to say, "I need your help. We need to plant the seeds at home now."

Even though I knew she wouldn't hesitate, my anxiety is immediately relieved by Kathleen's response. "I got it. You know I love a garden. And I would do anything for Cabooh. You, not so much, but Cabooh, anything. Same for Tim [Kathleen's husband]. Just give me the instructions and we will get it going."

CHAPTER 30
ENERGY AND HARMONY

Wilson is becoming restless, but I don't think it's due to the laid-back vibe of Kauai. He is hell-bent on getting back before New Year's Eve. I agree to his early departure, not because I want him to party with his friends, but because I'm suddenly questioning my judgment about bringing him out here in the first place. What kind of mom brings her son to assist with his baby sister's radical, detoxing seizure battle? Apparently, I'm the kind. But I also had hopes that Hawaii would in some way heal Wilson, too. I won't know if this bright-eyed, sober Wilson is here to stay until I let him go. So, I change his flight, pay the change fee, and let him leave.

Six days later, Jeff, Caroline, and I fly back together. I am confident that the long flight, the fatigue, and the cabin pressure will cause seizures. I prepare myself. But as we exit the second and final flight, I am in disbelief. No drugs and still *no seizures*. I feel like a winner.

But I'm only one member of the winning team. The biggest champion is the young girl who never once complained or asked for anything else to eat. This victory is possible because of the support of Billy and then Mike, the understanding from Holly, Wilson's devotion, Jeff's sacrifice and knowledge, his mentor's constant communication, the specialist, and now Kathleen and Tim. Pulsing with giddy energy, I want to dance off the airplane with a megaphone chanting, *seizure-free, seizure-free, our girl is seizure-free!*

As we descend the escalator into the Atlanta airport, there waiting are Mike and his mother. As soon as I see his face, I want to toss my suitcase into the air and rip off my clothes to get closer to the feeling of his chest against mine. I restrain myself, a little.

"Jeff, hold onto Caroline," I warn. I loop her arm into his and as soon as my foot hits the tile floor, I dart toward Mike. As I slip off my coat and let it fall to the ground, my arms fling around Mike's ribcage. With my face pressed into his neck, I allow my scalp to loosen its grip on my skull, teaching myself to breathe again.

On the drive home, we discuss the plan. Jeff tells us exactly what type and where to buy the clay in Athens. He is clear: "Don't tell them you plan to eat it. They may not sell it to you. Just act like a potter."

I belly laugh at this, "And what do potters act like? Is there an archetype I can study? Shall I buy some overalls and channel my best Demi Moore vibe?" And then I sway my shoulders as I break into the lyrics of "Unchained Melody" by The Righteous Brothers. As I hit the finale of the chorus, Mike's mom laughs. This fully German *frau* has no idea what we are talking about, but she can hear. She has just learned that I sing like a freshly castrated goat.

Jeff just says, "Oh, Tulip." I love when he calls me Tulip.

As we drive down the street toward home, I can see it. Tim and Kathleen have started the wheatgrass garden in the side yard, to the left of the house. Gratitude swells into my pores. Mike and his mom head into the house. Jeff and I get out of the car and walk Caroline straight to the garden. It's roughly an eight-by-fifteen-foot patch of barely-budding grass. Jeff puts his arm around Caroline and tells her, "Look Caroline. This is your wheatgrass. You can keep healing. I brought enough for about four more days. By then, this will still be kind of new, but you will be able to eat it."

He walks over to the bag of Black Kow manure-soil that Tim and Kathleen left partially used. "This is great. All organic. It's perfect. Now all we have to do is keep it going." He takes Caroline into the house to prepare her meal after the ten-hour trip.

I stay in the little garden, sitting down on our old regular grass and gently brushing my open palm across the budding wheatgrass. I smell the sweetness and feel its life force. What a miracle. From the dirt, on this tiny speck on our planet in Watkinsville, Georgia, we had what Caroline needed all along. We only had to listen to Mother Earth. Not doctor after doctor. I don't believe toxic pills can heal us. They block symptoms, fooling us into believing they are a cure. But they merely ease our pain while our body works with whatever nature we afford it to heal itself.

Sitting in the dirt at the edge of this baby garden, I am grounded by something I have never experienced. I feel fully alive and blanketed with peace. As my eyes close, I inhale the grassy aroma and imagine the earth's energy propagating from my core. The ground beneath me feels strong, like it's delivering the earth's vitality to keep me lively and fuel my diligence.

But before I open my eyes, I see something stronger than I could ever be; I see the love that surrounds us. I see the village of family and friends who are committed to helping Caroline claim a life of new dreams. While I once decided to never give anyone the power to break my spirit, I realize, when we relinquish control, we give people the power to make our spirits soar. It is community and the acceptance of help that are fortifying my ability to journey onward. Carrying its energy and peace with me, I walk out of the garden and into the arms of Team Caroline.

CHAPTER 31
TEAM CAROLINE EXPANDS

Jeff is adamant about using well water, and it must be transported in glass. He says the chlorine in city water will dilute the power of the clay and anything but glass could be a contaminant. Fortunately, Wilson has plenty of friends who live out in the country, and they are happy to transport their water to us. I start to object and say that we will retrieve it, but I catch myself and accept the help with deep gratitude. Not only will Caroline drink the water, but I need it for soaking and sprouting the wheat seeds and boiling and mixing the clay. In a matter of 24 hours, the first batch of sprouted wheat is done. I will continue to soak just enough wheat each night for the next day.

My next job is to "act like a potter" and buy the clay from a pottery studio. I must have nailed the role because buying it was easy. Preparing it is another story. Prepping the clay is the process I never saw in Kauai, because Jeff brought it to us every day, ready to consume. It's purchased as a 25-pound, rock-hard block of minerals that we have to break down and boil. We keep mixing it with well water until it looks like a Wendy's Frosty. It demands both time and strength. I feel consumed by this chore until the German engineer on Team Caroline intervenes.

I pull into the driveway after work and see that Mike is there. He's just outside the garage, wearing his safety goggles, hunched over a five-gallon bucket. An orange extension cord runs from the garage out to where he has both hands on the handle of a massive drill-like machine that is plunged down into the bucket. It's shaking his arms and shoulders as he keeps its neck upright and steady. The bobbing contraption gets louder as I walk closer, so I start to yell over it to inquire. But just as I open my mouth, I see.

He stops, turns off the machine, and looks up to kiss me. His glasses, his face, his clothes, are all splattered with taupe-colored goop. He has mixed the entire block of clay into a smooth, shiny supply of the pudding-like stuff that is helping Caroline to be without seizures for the first time in more than six years. He tries again to kiss me, but his lips just graze my front teeth, because I can't rein in my smile.

"Don't just stand there, my woman," he admonishes with a grin. "Get your ass in the house, out of those clothes, and let's make our girl her dinner."

I don't move but inquire, still beaming, "What the hell, Germany? What is that thing?"

"It's a cement auger," he answers as if he believes he is stating the obvious.

I bounce into the house and skip up the stairs. I'm in love with this man who keeps showing up, taking care of problems for which I assumed had no solution. I toss my navy slacks and pink blazer on the bed and look for my best mud-mixing attire for the evening.

I remember the last time I arrived home from work and found Mike in my garage. It was not quite a year ago, at the height of my delivery season. He knew that I was spending every evening digging through big storage buckets and boxes, in order to load my Expedition for the next day. I had to sort through a wide selection of graduation caps and gowns, memory books, T-shirts, hoodies, joggers, tassels, order forms, display items, and more.

My Germany was not impressed with the haphazard way I unloaded and reloaded each evening. But he never mentioned it; he just solved it. On that unforgettable afternoon, I pulled into the driveway, looked into the garage, and froze. With mouth agape, I stared. Mike heard me pull in, but he kept working for another minute. When he began to wonder why I hadn't opened the car door, he walked over and opened it for me.

He leaned down as if to check for a heartbeat and saw my face all screwed up with tears and a quivering lip. "What is it, woman? What's wrong? You don't like it?"

I gulped in air and chirped out, "I love it."

He pulled me out of the car and into his arms. "Then don't cry. Hey. It's not that big of a deal."

Oh, the hell it wasn't. My inventory no longer covered the floor. This man, my Germany, he completely transformed the garage so that I could identify products at a glance. Everything was organized by color, category, style, and size, stored neatly on shelves that were tailor-built to match the size of the storage bins and boxes.

This memory tingles my spine as I identify my least cute sweatshirt and leggings. I'm rummaging through my closet to find an old pair of forgotten running shoes as I ask myself, *why? Why has this man chosen me?*

He never explains it, he just keeps showing up with evidence of his love. I'm starting to believe it could last. I see that my journey as a mother does not deaden my ability to love a partner. As mothers, our children's suffering need not translate into a belief that we must put love on hold. Romantic love can fill us with a strength and joy that we can burgeon and return to our loved ones as well as our lover. That's why; that's why me.

I dash back down the stairs, grab a cold iced tea out of the fridge and follow the orange cord across the garage and over to Mike. I hand him the tea and he hands me the handle atop the cement mixer.

"Hold 'er steady, woman," he barks after a gulp of the cold drink. He hits the power button and suddenly my whole body is powering into healing my girl. My arms vibrate as I watch the smooth, shiny mud swirl around the bucket. Before the clay gets mixed with the wheatgrass, it deceptively looks like homemade ice cream. But it's better than ice cream. It's miracle minerals.

We get into a rhythm through the mild Georgia winter. Jeff shows me how much grass, grain, water, and clay to put in the Vitamix. Kathleen and Tim show up without fail, to keep the garden tilled, wheat planted, and new wheatgrass always available. Mike makes sure there is plenty of mud mixed and stored in airtight, glass containers. Friends continue to deliver well water with giving hearts. My duties are to keep wheat seeds freshly sprouted and to water and harvest the grass.

Lingering in the garden everyday becomes a ritual I crave. I chew a few blades of wheatgrass while the birds collaborate. The wind gently jostles the shrubs as a sweet, earthy scent makes me feel both grounded and light. The simple process of snipping the grass and placing it in the bowl is a centering melody. After trimming, I nourish the garden with water and listen to the gentle calling. In this little sanctuary, I don't resist my desire to languish. It is gratifying to nurture the garden that exists only to give. With gratitude, the last thing I do is brush my palm over a rich patch of grass, stand, and walk away.

The flame inside me now flickers with harmony, sending me back into the house with fresh clarity. I'm no longer at war, frantically fighting to an end, but courageously living out a journey where I embrace the challenges and the treasures just as they exist in each of life's minutes.

CHAPTER 32
YUM

Outside the wheatgrass garden, life keeps firing challenges our way. The peaceful routines I try to maintain for Caroline are challenged every day by sights, sounds, and aromas—the ding of the microwave, the smell of pizza, or the rustle of a bag of chips.

We all try to hide our food from Caroline. It feels cruel to eat in front of her, but to never eat in her presence is unrealistic. Because she hasn't tasted anything but earth, plant, and water in many weeks, her sense of smell is heightened. So rarely does a day pass when Caroline doesn't simply remark, "That smells so good."

When we left for Hawaii, Caroline was in a state of torment that was textbook drug addiction, from what I had read. I also attributed her trance-like state to drugs, not brain damage. We are past the 30-day mark on this diet and she has not had one seizure or one pill. This is the longest she has gone without a seizure since this journey began, more than six years ago.

But we are still waiting for her to come back to life fully. She has forgotten basic vocabulary words. She tries to pet squirrels, as if they are friendly puppies. When I try to explain that squirrels are not pets, she asks, "What is a squirrel?" And then the very next day, we will have the same conversation.

Today Jeff is leaving to go back home to Kauai. We don't need him to keep the project going; we have that mastered. But each day he has been giving Caroline massages, listening to her, and taking her for walks. His capacity for slowly repeating himself is limitless. Caroline seems to twinkle in the presence of her Uncle Jeff, and she looks forward to their daily interactions. I am panicked about her reaction to the news that it's time for him to leave. I think she will burst into tears or revert back into depression. But she doesn't cry, object, or express sadness. She just accepts the news with no emotion at all.

This perplexes and concerns me more than it relieves me. Her hair is finally regaining its sheen, her skin glows like it did when she was 12, and she once again smiles with her eyes. But her mind, her emotions, her intellect—they all seem stuporous. I can't believe epilepsy has caused such significant damage. But if not epilepsy and not drugs, why is Caroline still spaced-out and lacking emotion? I think she's hungry, needs more substance. But then I remember the people who live on this diet for many years and are vital and thriving.

After 40 days of only wheatgrass and clay, I ask Jeff about the future. I want to know how long he thinks we should keep this up. Could Caroline be healed? When will her cognitive deficit be repaired? And how about her weight? When she bends over, I can see her tail bone. Although her seizures, depression, and anxiety are gone, her ability to process and communicate is significantly diminished.

Jeff feels confident that her brain is still healing from years of being drugged and having seizures. Healing takes energy, which leaves the brain with little resources to perform to its full potential. He thinks that if she were to go back on medication and eat a typical American diet, her sensory processing and executive function would improve, because the energy that is being consumed by healing would be freed up for cognitive activity. But I'm concerned about the lack of progress from the clear damage done. So, we agree that it's time to transition into phase two: a vegan, organic, raw diet. She can continue to heal while slowly returning to more diverse foods.

Caroline has been watching the same six movies since she was 12. She has watched them so many times that the rest of us have them memorized. She can't seem to comprehend new stories or movies and I imagine there must be something soothing about watching the same stories over and over. This evening, *Freaky Friday* is playing as I walk into the den. I interrupt with, "Caroline, Honey, come into the kitchen. It's time for your dinner."

She slowly turns her face from the screen up to me and asks, "Sorry, what Mom?"

I repeat the request and she replies, "Can I wait until this is over?" She knows exactly what will happen and how mother and daughter, played by Jamie Lee Curtis and Lindsay Lohan, switch back into their own bodies and become a happy family. Yet she wants to finish this movie.

I entice her with, "The dinner is not wheatgrass. I think you will want to pause the movie for this meal."

She lets that statement register, looks back at the screen, and watches Jamie Lee Curtis pout like a 16-year-old. She glances back at my face. I smile, nod, and tell her again, "That's right. It's not wheatgrass."

Caroline is intrigued and forgets to stop the scene. While she slowly rises from the sofa, I watch Lindsay Lohan eat a French fry as if it's her hot, new lover.

Caroline walks into the kitchen with questions. "What is the food? Did you ask Uncle Jeff? Is it okay with Uncle Jeff?"

I assure her that this meal is his recommendation.

She sits down at the table and in front of her, I place a family-sized bowl filled with organic spring mix and eight raw Brazil nuts.

"Go ahead," I tell her, smiling. I can see she is not sure how to approach this new delicacy. "You don't need a spoon. Take a few bites of the lettuce and then have a nut. Just make sure you take your time and chew it very well."

I can see she doesn't understand. I think back to when she first came out of the coma at Egleston Children's Hospital. She couldn't remember how to chew or swallow.

Three times I repeat these instructions, and I demonstrate by taking a few bites myself.

She takes a bite of the lettuce, chews a bit, swallows and says, "Yum."

She then picks up a Brazil nut and bites off half of it. She chews and says nothing before she puts the other half in her mouth and keeps eating. I watch her eat. It's like watching a prisoner of war eat her first meal after being released back into freedom. She is aware of nothing other than the taste on her tongue and the feeling of chewing food. With more gusto than Lindsay Lohan and her French fry, she eats faster, as if she's racing. As she picks out the last few straggling pieces of spinach, she asks, "Can I have some more?"

CHAPTER 33
CHASING QI

During the first three years of trying to build my business, I learned to live with disappointment, but I never accepted it. After every losing presentation or rejection, friends and colleagues would tell me it wasn't my fault. They blamed the competitor, the committee, or the gutless nature of the decision-maker. These comments are what I never accepted. To blame my failures on factors beyond my control would have left me powerless, hopeless.

So, I blamed myself. I took responsibility, inspecting what I could have done differently. Looking back on those years of disappointment, I see it as suffering that wasn't wasted. I learned how to improve and I am now sharing the knowledge gained from my failures with ambitious new sales reps.

Be it the challenges of business or the hurdles of life, I reject the notion of a victim's mentality. It suffocates me. I don't think *why me* or *poor me*. I prefer to accept challenges as opportunities to be better built for battle. What I focus on, and hope will one day be of inspiration to others, is my response to agony. Heartache should not be wasted. To idle in pity would be to waste my suffering on the curdled soul of a victim. I want to model courage and stamina in such a way that perhaps it says to someone else, *I too can shed tears and fight for change while at the same time free myself to welcome love and experience happiness. If I can do this, the heartache will have been salvaged for joy.*

I'm sitting at a lunch table, inside the Morgan County High School cafeteria, taking graduation orders with my team. Yelling, laughing, silverware clanging, trays stacking, and chairs scraping along the tater-tot-littered floor all crowd my eardrums. In front of me is a long line of high school seniors waiting to place their orders and walk away with a bag full of items that prove their senior status. They buy T-shirts with smug phrases, tassels to hang in the cars their parents bought them, and travel mugs that we all know they are putting vodka in on the weekends.

As I rush through orders, I delight in this high school moment with each student. The next young lady steps up, I greet her, and she places her order in front of me. I begin to review and process it while she starts clicking messages into her cell phone with her French manicure. I reach for my calculator and while I can't hear my phone, I see that it's ringing. My hands freeze. I have to answer it. It's Miss Sharon, our new caregiver.

I look up at the young senior and say, "I'm so sorry, this

is my daughter's caregiver. She knows not to call during these hours unless it's urgent. Will just be a minute. I know you need to get to class."

She replies, "It's okay. My teacher doesn't care if we're late." She goes back to tapping on her phone screen.

I snatch up my phone and open it, "Miss Sharon? Is everything okay?" I ask, yelling over the cafeteria clamor.

In her slow, very southern drawl she replies, "I think so. Caroline was so tired when I brought her home. She lay down on the couch and before I knew it, she was on the carpet, having a seizure. She seems okay. But she won't get off the floor. So I didn't know if I should call someone, or what to do."

I keep holding the phone to my ear, but I can't speak. The lunch bell rings. The kids who were in my line have moved to the other two lines, stressing about getting to class on time. The one lackadaisical senior is still standing in front of me, enthralled with her phone. My head starts pounding to the speed of defeat.

I finally speak: "She's breathing, right?"

"Oh yes, or I would have called 911," Miss Sharon confirms.

"Sharon, this is called postictal state," I explain. "Just stay with her. Don't force her to get up, because she could fall. I will be out in my car in fifteen minutes. I will call you back then. Just sit tight, okay?"

My team helps me pack up and load the Expedition in record time. I thank them and without going back to the front office and talking with my customers, I'm gone. I am supposed to stop by one more school and discuss a workshop for student leaders. But I simply grip the wheel and head home. I wonder, *why am I so shocked? Caroline has slowly been weaning off the wheatgrass. Did I really believe it had cured her?* But then I get hopeful and think maybe she ate something processed or fried or sweetened or something.

I call Miss Sharon and drill her about Caroline's food. Nothing. No deviation from the piles of organic greens, nuts, soaked wheat, and well water.

As I drive, I will my emotions to sit down. Here are the facts: First, I know Caroline can't stay on the wheatgrass diet forever and live a full life. Second, the diet stopped her seizures, but she is still more confused than ever. And third, the slightest deviation from the diet seems to cause a seizure.

We will stay the course.

And we do. Ever so slowly, we introduce real food. And ever so slowly, the seizures return.

I'm standing in the center of the dried-up wheatgrass beside our house. It's showing some signs of life again, because spring comes early in Georgia. I feel peace out here. I'm about to sit down when I feel my phone vibrate from my pocket.

Shit. I need to leave this thing in the house when I walk out here to the wheatgrass sanctuary. It's messin' with my qi—the vital life force of my breath. I see a number I don't recognize, assume it's a customer on their personal phone, and answer, "Hello. This is Tara Heaton."

I hear a woman's voice. "Is this Mrs. Heaton, Wilson Heaton's mother?"

My qi drains and I confirm it is me.

"Your son is quite possibly one of the most talented writers to have ever been in my classes." My heart expands and smiles a bit.

She continues, "Making a call like this is not something I would typically do. But in this case, I just can't see letting such potential die without giving it a second chance. You see, Wilson missed the exam this morning. I would have excused it, had he called or emailed to explain. But I can't reach him. I will let him take the exam sometime before the end of the week. As I said, I don't normally do this, but I can't see letting him fail this class when I know he is an extraordinary writer. If he can email me today and schedule a make-up time, he should pass the class easily. Even with his missed assignments, he has an 88 average because, as I said, his work is exceptional."

She goes on to say she hopes he is safe and we hang up. I turn the phone over and over in my hand. My mind ping pongs as I dial his number.

No answer. Voicemail is full. I dial again. He picks up, clearly not awake, "Hel—" he clears his throat, "Hello."

I tell him what the professor said. I want a reassuring explanation, but here is what I get:

"I'm sorry. Mom, I'm sorry, I overslept."

It is 3 p.m. Right now, my son, who is genetically gifted to connect to people, to excel in sports, to write, to climb, is giving it all away for his one true love—adrenaline. Drinking, smoking, music, parties, dancing, laughing, danger, and sex.

I think back to when I was in college. I kept a job. I went to my classes and passed them. And, I partied plenty. In exactly four years, I earned a diploma and tossed a cap in the air. I was running toward something. I wanted to have a career, because it would give me freedom, challenge me, and energize me. I don't see Wilson running toward anything. He is running *from* something.

"Wilson. Call the professor right now. She is giving you a chance that you don't deserve. Get your ass out of whoever's bed you are in and go grab this chance. This could be your last one. If you fail out again, no other college will take you. And I promise you this, even if they did, I won't be paying for it."

He mumbles something that sounds like a commitment. I snap the phone shut and toss it into the grass. Trying to reclaim my qi, I crawl my hands across the earth and remain in downward dog pose, but I know it's a joke. All I can think about is how I am supposed to be helping Wilson. I can choose to believe it's on him now. But clearly, he isn't capable. I see him running and I have to admit, I also see where he learned it. Even if he were at a place malleable to adopting the behavior of a parent, he isn't here to notice the change in me. He can't see that I have slowed down, taken time to soften, to cry, to feel.

As I walk back into the house, Holly drives up, windows open, rapping in sync with Nicki Minaj. Apparently, my little girl has heard this tune a time or two. I keep staring, wondering when Holy Holly left the building. She keeps singing, bopping her head until she finishes her crude sing-along, and then cuts off the car and climbs out from behind the wheel. I grab her face, smooch her cheek, and say, "That music is disgusting."

She tries to shut the car door, but I grab it and peer into the little black Jetta that her dad used to drive. Diet Coke bottles, lip gloss, T-shirts, Dairy Queen spoons, papers, shoes, French fries, grocery sacks, CDs, textbooks, notebooks, jackets, Pop-Tart wrappers, pens, nail polish . . . oh, you get the picture.

"Unacceptable, Holly."

She starts telling me that she is convinced she has ADHD and she is going to clean it out, but my cell phone once again intervenes.

I talk to my customer while I watch Holly, in full-snit mode, grab wads of trash from her car. She chunks garbage into the bin as if she's trying to punish the innocent remnants of chaos. As I end the call, I can't help but chuckle a little, which makes her even bitchier. And then, I just can't help it, I start laughing.

"What?" she yells. "Why are you laughing? I have a lot going on. I'm just oh so soooorry that I don't have time to properly clean my car!"

I cover my mouth with my hand, because I can't kill the laughter. I bear down and compose myself enough to speak. "Honey. You do realize, I did not put that trash in your car. Yet somehow, you are mad at me because the inside of your car looks like it belongs to a high school hoarder."

She is not amused. "Well instead of laughing, you could help me. You don't know how busy I am. I have to be back at school for DECA and then a Beta Club meeting. And I have three days left to sell that gift wrap for cheerleading. And I have a paper due tomorrow. And I have to work tomorrow and Friday so I have no more time. And! Everyone else's mom helps them! I am doing this all by myself. I have no help! I want to get tested for ADHD. I need Adderall!"

I dismiss the mom slam, the request for prescription drugs, and zero in on the finish line. I cling to the three more days until spring break. "Holly, three more days, baby. Let's remember where we are going in only three more days."

I hug my baby girl and leave her in the driveway. Even though Holly is excelling, I know she is hurting. It doesn't disable her like it seems to be doing to Wilson. No, it's doing something else. She is screaming to be seen. She watches her parents frantically race to the needs of her older siblings. This is teaching her that trauma produces love. I don't want that to be the single theme of her memories, or to define her behavior for the future. I want to show her that, not in spite of our journey, but because of it, we have the capacity to be drenched in joy. After all, Holly is the one who first cautioned me not to waste life minutes.

I think back to December, her sixteenth birthday party . . . the one that I promised would include some unknown magical surprise. It did. She opened her card from Mom.

242

Inside were two airline tickets to LaGuardia and a little note: *New York City, my angel. You and me. Five days to light up the city, just the two of us. Happy Birthday to the little light of my life. I simply . . . adore you. Love, Mom.*

I'm so excited about making this memory with Holly. I have been telling her that New York is nothing like LA, where we'd gone for Caroline's biofeedback. New York is real and raw. It's a place where stockbrokers, artists, bartenders, designers, performers, and all-out dreamers are hustling. It feels like an endless flashmob where each dancer is chasing a marker that is theirs alone. It's a contagious energy. You either keep up or get out of the way.

CHAPTER 34

POTPOURRI

Some choices we question and some we just know deep in our soul that, no matter the cost, it's the right call. Taking my baby girl to New York was undoubtedly a good call. It was like one of those dreams that make you sad to wake up.

At the start of our trip we agreed, we needed to see the site of what was once the World Trade Center. After bagels and coffee, we walked quickly in the cold, gloved-hand in gloved-hand. As we approached the crowd, our pace slowed. Massive fences guarded the space where the Twin Towers that housed exhilarating careers for thousands had become just two canyons in Lower Manhattan. We stepped up, and we looked down.

Without words, we let go of our clasped hands, tugged off one glove, and quickly locked our two bare hands back together. We stood staring in silence as minutes passed before Holly took her free hand to brush away a tear. She glanced over at me, back at the pit in the earth, and said:

"One minute, someone's mom was right here, sitting at her desk, talking on the phone with her daughter. And the next minute, she was gone."

I lifted her soft hand to my lips and kissed her cold knuckles. We peered down into the motionless, dark abyss and then up into the bright blue sky with the traveling clouds.

Holly continued, "Almost three thousand people were right here living out their last life minutes. I wish they could have known."

As we strolled away, Holly asked, "What would you do, Mom? If you knew you were living your last minutes, what would you do?"

Without considering the crowd and where they were all racing to be, I stopped, took her face in my hands, and kissed her damp cheek.

"This, Honey. This is how I would be spending my last life minutes–celebrating life with you, your brother, and your sister."

Each day of our trip was fueled by the energy of the city and the retreat from reality. I watched two cheeks that remind me of Rainier cherries turn up to the sky. The golden-brown eyes glistened as the spirit of a six-year-old emerged.

New York was learning the difference between the pretense of happiness and visceral joy. The pretense of happiness is to fight off grief. It is classic toxic positivity, born of the dogmatic message: *Smile Honey, things could be so much worse.* The pretense of happiness would have been to prance around New York with Holly, feigning cheerfulness, but consumed in my own thoughts.

But visceral joy—it is the acceptance of grief. To have joy is to embrace the energy of pain, repurpose it, and pour it into the treasure of the moment. Joy is intention. Joy is our fighting spirit. New York was joy.

Tired but energized, we arrive home from our trip and walk into the den to find Wilson, Caroline, and a dog named Sandy. I hug and smooch Caroline, but I'm staring at Wilson and back down to this sallow-blond, 40-poundish potluck of a dog. She's maybe a Chihuahua, Chow, Collie, Labrador, Husky mix.

Wilson comes at me with his signature enthusiasm: "Mom! Sandy is a seizure dog. She can detect seizures. I got her for Caroline!"

I shake my head a little to make sure I'm seeing and hearing correctly.

"Wilson, these dogs cost thousands of dollars. They are highly trained and very hard to come by. Where did you get her and what's the catch?"

"There is no catch, Mom," he assures me. "This guy gave her to me. I told him about Caroline and he said I could have her."

I wonder what I'm missing and don't know what to ask first. If this scruffy-looking dog can detect seizures and if Caroline would come out of this damn trance, then we are looking at a real safety solution. Caroline's seizures have slowly returned. But the more maddening thing is that her awareness and cognition are still significantly diminished. I have read enough about seizure service dogs to know that the epileptic and the dog must bond. I'm starting to worry that Caroline will never return to us. She pays no attention to Sandy. She's not even smiling at her brother. She is just staring at the television. But the television is off. I settle in beside her, and the story unfolds.

Wilson plans to take care of Sandy the seizure dog. He never went back to take that exam and it seems he has decided that college is not for him. He is going to work on farms and keep riding bulls until he is invited to go on the road. He says he is not cut out for college and that he will be the next Tuff Amos, a bull-rider phenomenon. But until his bull-riding skills and nomad spirit are rewarded, the grand news is that Wilson is going to take care of Sandy, because he is back home to live.

Sandy the seizure dog has no interest in Caroline. She only has a heart for Wilson. She is like an itchy ottoman that you don't really notice until you trip over it. But in her defense, Caroline makes zero effort. In another life, I know I would have fallen head over heels for this docile canine. But Sandy is a subtle yet constant reminder that the Caroline who was once unable to resist any dog, is gone. For now.

We stay the course. I keep feeding Caroline organic everything, nothing processed, no sugar, no refined oils, no flour, no acid, and no dairy. I have returned some clean, lean protein to her diet slowly, along with whole grains, and massive plates full of organic greens several times a day. She has gained enough weight so that I can't see her tailbone through her sweatpants. The seizures are returning, but her cognition isn't.

I'm standing in the kitchen, right in the place where I have danced with the humans I love most on earth. Mike is with me, telling me that he got the official offer for the career move of his dreams, and plans to move to the thriving little city of Greenville, South Carolina. It's an easy two-hour drive north. With his current job, he is gone to Asia for weeks at a time, so this doesn't feel like a tough stretch for us.

Mike is helping me fix food for everyone else and get Caroline's meal prepared first. Her plate is ready. I have disposed of the pasta box and marinara sauce jar, and I have hidden the salad dressing and the baguette with a towel.

"We ready for Caro to eat?" Mikes asks. I nod and he walks into the den to tell her it's time for her dinner. He returns to the stove beside me and continues cooking his German meat dumplings. As I sauté onions, I return a call to my new sales associate regarding his presentation tomorrow. I offer some suggestions as I add mushrooms and garlic to the onions. We agree on the perfect story arc, so I end the call, pick up Caroline's plate, and turn to take it to her at the table.

I am not sure I believe what I see. She is already eating. She is making a face because it is hard to chew potpourri. I race the four steps to her side and almost slide down onto my knees.

"Oh, Honey, no!" My voice is desperate. "That's not your dinner. That's the bowl of potpourri that we keep on the table for decoration."

Her eyes squint and her brow furrows with confusion.

"Spit that out. Spit it out! Open your mouth. Like this, ahhh."

She slowly opens her mouth and I say, "Wider. That's right. Like me. Ahhhhh."

She dramatically opens her mouth to capacity, and I use my fingers to scrape dark pink bark off her tongue.

"Spit. Into my hand."

I wipe her stained saliva onto the Ann Taylor slacks I have been meaning to change out of.

"Here, Honey. Here is your dinner. This. This is your dinner," I assure her as I get off my knees and rub her boney back.

As she begins to eat again, I turn to Mike. With four more steps back across the kitchen, I aim to fall into his arms. But my heartache burns through to my legs, and I melt down into the tile floor. My chest heaves in and I let the agony flood out. My daughter, she is four feet away from me, but she is gone. I want to vomit out the grief, to stop missing her. I see her. But it's merely her shell, a cruel reminder of who she once was, and who she planned to be, a second-grade teacher and a mom. That's what she asked for from this life. She asked to care for children. That was it. And this heinous affliction has taken that from her.

I hear Wilson and Holly walk in, ready for spaghetti and meat dumplings.

"What's wrong? What happened? What's wrong with Mom?"

Mike pulls me from the floor and I grip the sleeve of his shirt. He holds onto me and says, "Your mom is just having a hard day."

I steady my feet, suck in oxygen, and pull away.

"Mayo Clinic," I say. "That's what's next. We are going to Rochester. I hear they are on the cutting edge for epilepsy. This diet is over."

I stand erect. "That's right. We are going to the Mayo Clinic. That's where this war on seizures is taking us next."

Mike kisses my head and I softly smile. "Caroline?"

She looks up from her spinach and kale.

"How would you like some spaghetti for dinner?"

CHAPTER 35
UNDEFEATED

W e aren't scheduled for the Mayo Clinic until the following year, in February 2011. So we retreat back to Emory and get Caroline on a new cocktail of AEDs. She is a little bit more aware lately; I assume because even though her seizures have returned, they are milder than before the wheatgrass diet, and she's consuming foods that trigger excitatory neurotransmitters. But the awareness comes with a price.

The misery is also slowly returning, along with a new challenge. She obsesses. She is obsessed with her weight gain, her tan, and her hair. And she is obsessed with Holly. She compares herself to Holly, hyper-focused on anything her younger sister can do or have that she cannot: a car, a job, sleepovers, cheerleading. These obsessions materialize as relentless questions. Obsession mixed with short-term memory loss is a maddening trap. We are in survival mode until we can get to Rochester next year. This means surviving December and the holidays.

Christmas comes every single year. If it were every third year, or even every other year, I would have a better attitude about it. But shit, by the time you recover, you're planning it all over again. And now I don't even have Billy to decorate the house anymore! This year I think I have figured out a way to skip Christmas. I still can't believe Mike, Billy, and Channing all agreed, but it's all planned. Mike and I, Billy and Channing, Mike's son Konrad, Wilson, Caroline, and Holly are going on a cruise to the Bahamas over Christmas. The community around me is decorating, baking, shopping, wrapping—and stressing. Meanwhile, I feel like I have a dirty little secret. I'm just making sure we can all show up with flip flops, sunscreen, and passports.

It's the first day out to sea and we all gather to find a family spot by the pool. But Wilson and Holly are not interested in family bonding. They are working the deck like it's a political rally. I'm used to Wilson and his meet-no-stranger vibe.

But I'm watching Holly flirt with some guy who has long blonde hair. When did she get so thin? It appears she has used her Your Pie job money to buy new swimsuits, which are not made for swimming. These are tiny bikinis that conceal only what's necessary to make them legal. She sways about the deck, playfully laughs with a hair toss, and languishes as she massages sun lotion into her legs and flat stomach.

I want to snatch her up by her hand, bring her over

to our chairs, play Yahtzee, and nibble French fries. Only Caroline is more fixated on Holly than me. She wants to join the young people gathered near the hot tub. But we know I will never again leave her side at a swimming pool. So I sit and try to explain to her why she can't, again and again and again. Mike tries to help, but with his German accent, she can't understand a word he says, so she looks back to me for interpretation.

The first excursion off the ship starts on a shuttle bus. Our party of eight leaves room for only four more passengers. We ride along on hot pleather seats, chattering nonstop. We laugh at memories from when the kids were little. Channing tells some stories about Billy not understanding gay protocol. We make plans for a family camping trip in Channing's new RV. And we decide to spend a weekend in Greenville as soon as Mike gets settled in the new house that will eventually be ours. We don't even notice how quiet the other four Christmas-skipping vacationers are until one of them speaks up from the front of the bus.

She literally raises her hand and says, "Can I ask y'all a question?" She doesn't wait for a reply. "How exactly are all of you related?"

We giggle and I speak up, pointing for clarity, "Well, this is my boyfriend. That's my ex-husband and that's his boyfriend. Those three are our children and he is my boyfriend's son."

The lady smiles a wide smile and says, "Wow. That's spectacular. You should write a book!"

The entire cruise vacation is not spectacular. On one of the last evenings, we are finishing dinner and Wilson has not shown up. I'm annoyed and disappointed.

"Can Caroline stay here with y'all?" I ask. I'm going to find Wilson.

I start charging through the ship like I'm looking for a toddler who fancies bars. First, I check the outdoor bars, then the night clubs. No sign of him. I quickly ascend the stairs to another pool with a large deck that has turned into a dance floor. Of course. And there he is, beer in the air, swaying, and chanting some pop-tune lyrics with 30 of his new best friends. I'm pissed that he missed dinner. But I can't help delighting in how he connects with people and soaks up life minutes like perhaps we all should. At some point, he sees me and beckons for me to join his party. I just laugh and wait.

When the song ends, he walks over and starts into one of his apologies, this one about missing dinner because he couldn't find his shoes. I realize he is drunk.

"Wilson, you need food," I tell him. "Let's go sit at the bar. You can get a burger and a Coke."

We sit and Wilson asks for a beer. I protest. He persists. I protest. The bartender brings the beer.

I turn to him, put my elbow on the bar, and put my chin in my hand. He devours the burger like he devours every-thing. He chugs the beer. I scoot the Coke closer. He chugs that, too.

He starts again with an apology. I tell him to forget about dinner and cheap flip flops as I dive into another rendition of the same speech, begging him to see that he is running from pain.

He interrupts, "Mom. I am fine. I just like to party. I wasn't meant for college. I need to be with nature and animals. It's where I feel most alive."

"You know I will support whatever you are passionate about, right?" I start. "I mean I put you on a plane to Kansas so you could go to rodeo school, for God's sake. But you are throwing away your potential by partying, using alcohol to cope with trauma and grief." I can't help myself. I can't stop this merry Christmas lecture. "Dealing with learning about your dad after your suspicions and—"

"Mom, forget about Dad and his gayness. I love Dad. If he's gay, I really don't care. It was just a shock. But—" and he stops.

In an instant, the party boy is gone, drained from his body. His lip quivers, he hunches over, puts his head in his hands, and barely cracks out one word: "Caroline."

And then I watch as his shoulders shake uncontrollably.

After what feels like a lifetime, he sits up, wipes his nose, and shudders his upper body back and forth, trying to shake off the hurt. He tries to explain, but his bottom lip objects, quivering again.

"Take your time," I say.

And then he speaks through sobs. "Why? Why did this happen to her? Is she ever going to get better, Mom? She lost everything. She's so innocent. Everyone loved her because she was just so fuckin', oh sorry, so, so sweet. This can never stop hurting." He heaves. He chokes. "Never."

I don't argue; I agree. I tell him he is right. "As long as you are alive to love Caroline, the heartache will never be gone." He looks stunned and I continue. "You are running from this, Wilson. Pain, it's undefeated. If you don't let yourself feel it, it will catch you and it will beat you."

As I explain to Wilson, I am reminding myself what I know. "You are in agony; your heart is not broken. It is aching, but heartache is not lethal. It is an energy that you can use to express yourself and make the world a sunnier place. Heartache is the source of our capacity to experience joy. You can't feel that right now because you are still trying to figure out how to fight it off. You can't win that fight."

When we return home from the cruise, I start to count down the days before we leave for Rochester in February. Caroline endures more seizures and is riddled with anxiety. I can't imagine taking this trip alone. But I don't have to imagine it; Billy and I plan to go together. It will be two weeks in snow and I know I will have to get out, move, and breathe hard, in order to give my best to our daughter. So I leave my office at four sharp to shop for warm, functional gear and get back home in time to let Wilson take my car to work.

As I drive home, I try to call Wilson, to make sure he is up and ready for work. No answer. Even though it's almost five, I know I will be trying to get him up and out the door to work on time. I call Mike. He is working and doesn't pick up. But I already know what he will say. Like a page out of an Al-Anon guidebook, he will tell me that as long as I support Wilson's habits, financially and otherwise, he will not change. He will say that I *enable* my son to continue down this dangerous path and there is only one way back up—from rock bottom. The words *You can't get up from death* shiver through me.

When I get home, Miss Sharon informs me that Wilson is in his bed. Habit starts to send me upstairs in a fury, but something stops me. It could be wisdom, it could be exhaustion, but I don't go. I bid Miss Sharon goodbye and start preparing a light meal.

Dinner is finished and cleaned up when Wilson stumbles in and plops himself down at the kitchen counter. He berates himself for missing work, waiting for me to disagree. I say nothing. I take his plate out of the microwave and sit in silence as he tries to eat black-eyed peas, rice, and broccoli. After a few bites, he takes out a pack of cigarettes and heads out the door. I follow him; we sit on the porch and I stare at my son. What my mind sees is the young man, hunched over the bar on that cruise, crying uncontrollably for his sister.

Still, I believe he has it in him to be the young man in Hawaii—alive, generous, clear, and strong. I tell him no more chances. He cannot live in this house if he can't keep his word, keep a job, and contribute. Somehow the conversation turns into how I can help Wilson course correct. He convinces me that a vehicle is the answer to his problems, an overall panacea to his current state of chaos. And of course, he has already found a vehicle, a little red truck. It's only a few thousand dollars. He just needs to *borrow* the money.

Love is strong, but our response to it can be a weakness. I have always seen action as the key to keeping hope alive, but perhaps restraint is also an action. The literary world borrowed a Greek term called *hamartia*, which is a character's tragic flaw. For me, and I think for so many mothers, love can also be our *hamartia*, that inability to sit by and let your child learn how strong they are, and grow their confidence by climbing out of shit on their own.

It was my *hamartia* that wrote a check for that truck. As soon as Wilson had wheels, he got something else that he felt he desperately needed—a dog. Wilson was gifted a chocolate lab puppy whom he named Tuff. Tuff Amos. Never in my life have I seen an animal-human connection like this duo. Wilson takes Tuff hiking, fishing, swimming, and as a tagalong when he is on a horse. He takes him to farms, practice arenas, and rodeos. I am starting to believe that Tuff is just the therapy Wilson needs.

CHAPTER 36
THE ANTIDOTE TO GLOOM

Finally. Billy, Caroline, and I prepare to leave for Rochester. Holly stays with Julie. Wilson, Sandy the seizure dog, and Tuff stay at the house.

A trip to the Mayo Clinic has been suggested to me many times. And many times, I have researched and rejected it because, in Caroline's unique case, the track record of traditional medical practitioners is poor. I assume that epileptologists from all the level-four epilepsy centers across the country attend the same conferences and are exposed to the same studies and findings. So my logic was that, unless we are looking at surgery, what more could the Mayo Clinic do?

With that, we went on a path toward natural and non-traditional healing. Of all those attempts, only one trial stopped the seizures—wheatgrass and clay. Even so, living on that diet is not sustainable and the fear around Caroline's cognition and processing was mounting.

So why Mayo now? If possible, my research intensified as we began to wean from the wheatgrass diet and return to drugs that only mitigate seizure activity. A recurring theme from Mayo Clinic patients was uncovered: The neurologists are devoted to seeing each patient as an individual case. They have a reputation for innovation—doing everything possible to create a plan specific and unique to each patient. This concept is foreign to us. It's as though other doctors have been trying to convince us to accept Caroline's fate. But if what I am reading is true, we may meet a team that won't take defeat easily.

As we sit with Caroline, watching the technician glue all the leads to her head, I wonder how healthcare systems can be so dramatically different. These Mayo Clinic people have their act together. A 1 p.m. appointment means 1 p.m. It's like Johns Hopkins, only happier. Each scrub team member seems as if they actually have a heart. Maybe it's due to acting classes, but I don't care. To be greeted on time and spoken to with kindness was an unexpected, refreshing antidote to my hospital anxiety.

Billy is on his break and it's my turn to sit with Caroline in her room and wait. It's the fourth time we have admitted her into the hospital, hooked her up to leads, monitors, and a video recorder, stopped her meds, and waited. We are waiting for seizures, so the doctors can analyze the origin of them and her brain activity. We know how this will go. When meds are pulled, the seizures come hard and strong. We sit and wait to witness what we have devoted over seven years of life to preventing.

No seizure has come yet. Caroline is talking non-stop, but I'm not really listening. I'm thinking about Billy and the thought of coming here and enduring this without him. Billy and I quickly get back into our tag team routine that we mastered so many years ago. We have one hotel room and there is a daybed in the room with Caroline. So, we take turns sleeping in a real bed and sleeping beside Caroline in the hospital. We take turns going for walks, getting air, taking calls, and showering.

For years before Billy and I split up, I wanted him out. Existing in a dead marriage felt like living in cold, gray clouds that never cleared for the sun. Our house was full, my work was rewarding, yet it was the only time in life I felt truly lonely. But now, being beside Billy is warmth, like a favorite blanket. The pain that used to encase his face has dissolved. He smiles with his eyes again.

Being Billy's confidant, friend, and partner in parenting is a treasure in this life. I hurt for divorced couples who are riddled with hate. I would say what we have is due to forgiveness, but there is nothing to forgive. We have something else, a rare kind of trust. We trust in each other's intentions and that we keep our word. I chose Billy as my family in 1989, and I still choose him as my family today.

Remembering a conversation Mike and I had right after he moved to Greenville makes me smile. We were out for an early-morning walk and I said, "Babe, this is a cool town. I love it. I love you. But still, I gotta have friends when I move here."

And Mike said, "You have friends. They can visit."

I laughed, "Yes, but you don't connect with my friends. I want us to have *our* friends. Which of my friends can you see as *our* friends?"

Mike paused. He thought. And then he said, "Billy."

I get it. I know why Mike likes Billy. It's summed up best by remembering back to a road trip that Kathleen, Tim, Billy, and I took years ago. Tim and Billy in the front seat, Kathleen and me in that back seat, chewing on Twizzlers and trying to juice up the conversation. I asked, "If y'all could be remembered for one thing after you are gone from this earth, what would it be?"

Tim probably joked and said, "a rich son of a bitch." Kathleen said she would be known for superior taste in music and beer. But I will never forget Billy's response. With little contemplation, he replied, "I would want people to say I was kind."

Man was I a hard-charging bitch back then. I remember thinking *how basic, how banal*. And today? I see that there is little else that matters than kindness. Kindness is a remedy for gloom. When we express kindness through actions or words, it makes someone else's world a bit lighter. So much of what we possess can be lost in an instant, but the ability to be kind can never be taken from us; it is ours to give without limits. Maybe these Mayo Clinic people are not acting. Maybe they offer kindness because we showed up with it first.

Billy walks back into the hospital room carrying two cups of coffee. He hands me one, sets his down, and wipes the melted snow from his short coat and jeans. I hug him.

After the coffee warms me and we chat with Caroline, I suit up in my down coat, scarf, hat, and gloves and leave for a hike through the little town of Rochester, Minnesota.

The whistle of the wind and the rhythm of my boots crunching in the snow let my mind wander free. I'm transported back to the years of escaping the torment of hospitals. With every one of Caroline's in-patient stays, I would find a hiding place where I could smoke a cigarette, curse the universe, and will myself to stay tough and mission driven. It was how I coped with being at the hospital, and with life.

The hospital experience hasn't changed. A heavy-hearted fatigue still renders me useless. My brain tells me to get some work done, but my emotions balk at the notion. Unless I'm tending to Caroline, I just stare into nothing. At the same time, the anxiety comes in waves, making my heart race, my breathing erratic. It gives me a frenzied, worthless energy like a lightning bug trapped in a mason jar. What has changed is my response to this experience. I don't fight it and I don't berate myself. I accept it and ride along.

As I return to Caroline's room, I see she is sleeping after what Billy says was a long, hard seizure. While he rests, I stand over Caroline and let the hurt in. As I immerse myself in the loss of the young girl I once knew, I taste sweetness. I lean down, close my eyes, and remember the 12-year-old girl with the willowy smile and the calm confidence. I remember the friends that used to gather up in her room. I remember how she was the serenity between the untethered energy of her brother and sister. I remember how she stood up for outcasts and underdogs. I remember her determination to conquer what didn't come easily.

I remember her dream: to be a second-grade teacher and a mom.

Between her gauze-wrapped head and the tape across her nose, I kiss a silky space on her cheek. It's still the same cheek, the same skin, a familiarity I want to inhale and preserve. I let my tears trickle down. The beeps and clicks of the monitors are now the familiar sound of my journey, a sporadic melody reminding me that freedom is in our response to what life hurls our way.

The two weeks at the Mayo Clinic affirmed what we have been told, but also helped us discover some new insight. We knew what they would find as a result of the seizures: Caroline is not a candidate for dissection surgery because her seizure origins are multi-focal. Yep, we knew this.

She also had an MRI, an fMRI, and a very extensive psyche evaluation. The results are tough to read. The official diagnosis has progressed to Lennox-Gastaut syndrome. This is a specific type of epilepsy that presents an abnormal EEG with seizures that worsen cognitive, emotional, and behavioral function. The IQ portion also shows significant decline that aligns with the diagnosis. The encouraging news is that there is minimal visible damage to Caroline's gray matter, which verifies a healthy brain and potential for healing. And so, if we can stop the seizures, there is a chance of regaining some of what has been lost.

The plan for seizure control is a new drug, Clobazam, that has been getting results for patients with Lennox-Gastaut epilepsy in Canada. Several studies show up to an 80-percent decline in seizures for people who have tried seven or more of the current AEDs. The side effects are nothing very different from most of the others. We can have the medication shipped from Canada directly to our mailbox.[5]

This news is soul-pumping energy. I want to go out and dance in Rochester's nine inches of snow. We are headed back home with a new plan, a new hit to our budget, and hearts bursting with hope.

---

[5] The medication brand name is Onfi, and the drug is Clobazam. This was before it was accessible in US pharmacies. It is now a very common AED in the US. It is, however, another addictive benzodiazepine.

CHAPTER 37
CAKE AND COMMITMENT

As the months tick by, Caroline improves. She is more alert and the seizures are mild and rare. We put the stroller away, which feels like a victory ceremony. I know that in time, this medication will be like the others and will run its course of efficacy. I am reminded of little Jack's parents in the TBI clinic, how they were overcome with gratitude for the bright side of the day. My heart celebrates every day that Caroline is able to live off the couch, engage with people, and find a reason to smile.

What used to be a ruthless fight for a seizure-free life has become a prevailing journey to help a now-20-year-old Caroline live as independently and fully as she can. I have not abandoned the war on epilepsy; I have accepted it as part of the life of Caroline's mom. I am learning to see this role as an honorable challenge that I have been awarded because, yes, I am a mother of a child with special needs. My respect for parents whose children require extraordinary care has exploded. I want to learn from them, lean on them, and help them if I am ever able. But right now, they are helping me. They are sharing resources, opportunities, programs, and policies that apply to Caroline. I am accepting and grateful. One day I will turn to a new mom of a child with special needs and pay it forward.

One of the resources shared is the most magical organization I have ever witnessed, Extra Special People (ESP), Inc., in Watkinsville, Georgia.[6] It's Friday night and I'm walking Caroline in the door to her first ESP outing, a pizza and painting party. She has been desperate to make friends, and so even the anticipation of this three-hour activity has transported her to a state of joy.

As we walk in, the greetings are plentiful and enthusiastic. Caroline is instantly immersed, introducing herself and smiling as if she is the star of the event. I flash back to watching her host her twelfth birthday party and I see that my daughter's spirit still reigns.

Other parents leave their children and almost dance back out the door toward a few hours of freedom. I too want to dance out that door, but I'm afraid of a seizure, a fall, and an injury. For the fourth time since I registered her for pizza and painting, I inquire, "Are you sure I shouldn't stay? Just in case she has a seizure?"

A young assistant introduces herself as Jordan. She puts her arm around me and gently guides me toward the door, saying, "Mrs. Heaton, several of these folks have

---

[6] ESP, Inc. is led by CEO Laura Whitaker and now has several locations and divisions. Caroline still attends the summer camp and it's still the most magical place on earth. Sorry, Disney World.

seizures. We are trained and equipped for them. Part of why we do this is for you. Go and enjoy yourself."

I glance back at Caroline one more time and see her smiling, chatting, being silly, and being accepted. She never looks toward me.

As I leave, I remember Loretta, and how, with the same gentle sweetness as Jordan, she guided me out of the TBI rehabilitation center on the first day eight years ago. I remember scrambling to my car for cigarettes. But tonight, I don't scramble; I drive slowly to Big City Bread in Athens and enjoy the sound of my two feet crunching across the gravel parking lot. From a cozy booth under a window, I order a piece of caramel walnut cake and a cup of chamomile tea. I savor the cake, sip the tea, and devour the moment. I am filled with admiration for the parents I'm meeting, with gratitude for Caroline's chance to make friends, and with love—love of a life I am creating, not despite the heartache, but because of it.

Caroline is doing so well that we plan for her to spend a weekend with her grandparents. It's a weekend in mid-November. Billy and Channing want to go out of town, they need a dog sitter, and Mike and I like the idea of a little weekend getaway to Atlanta. So, we will stay at their house. We can bring Mike's dog Wolfie and take care of Channing's German Shepherd, Montana. Bruiser died a few weeks back and Montana is rather depressed, so Wolfie is a playful distraction. Holly is a senior in high school and will stay home with her brother. Mike's son is with his mother. Except for dogs, Mike and I have a rare, romantic weekend, free and alone.

We walk the two huge dogs all morning. Then we leave them at home and enjoy nachos on a deck at a taqueria. I'm sitting across from Mike, nibbling on a tortilla chip and watching the crinkly eyes. I pull my foot out of its sandal, stretch out my leg, and tuck my toes under the inside of his thigh.

"Oh, *du kleiner flittchen*," Mike says with exaggerated shock.

I giggle. "I don't have on any panties."

"What would your mother say?" he asks.

"Oh, she would be delighted," I assure him.

He keeps smiling, sips his Diet Coke and says, "I want to marry you. I want to grow old with you. I want you to be my wife."

I was hoping to talk about the breeze under my skirt. But I see the desire behind the twinkle in those eyes. I hesitate. My hesitation is fear. I recoil at the thought of Mike wanting to leave one day, but staying out of duty or, even worse, pity.

I'm afraid marriage could make us lazy or ungrateful. In this moment, I'm simply afraid to lose this magic.

I used to cope by running. Today, I don't run. I look into the eyes that are like champagne for my soul, and I tell Mike the truth. I tell him why I'm afraid to get married and then say, "Maybe one day." He slides the chip basket aside; reaches for my hands and assures me he will wait for one day and he will be here even if one day never comes.

Mike and I are sound asleep at Billy and Channing's house when the phone rings. It's a little after 2 a.m. and I know it has to be Wilson. I snatch open the phone without looking at the number and grumble out a hello.

It's Holly. She is screaming, "Mom. You need to come home! Wilson called and I had to drive downtown to pick him up. He is wasted and he won't go to bed. Why am I dealing with this?"

As Mike and I drive home in the middle of the night, I know what I have to do. We don't discuss it. I just tell him. "I'm going to tell Wilson he has to leave. I will give him until December thirty-first. But tomorrow I will tell him that he has to move out."

Mike says nothing. He just drives and holds my hand.

CHAPTER 38
THE LAST PHONE CALL

Initially, I started studying the brain as Caroline's warrior. But somewhere along the way, I recognized all the ways I could apply what I was learning. My knowledge informed my work as a sales leader and speaker. Today, my family journey and the insight I have gained help me dissect human behavior, habits, and addiction. We humans create pleasure-seeking habits to cope with the barnacles of life. When we experience stress to any degree, the brain objects by seeking relief, reward, or escape.[7]

Wilson is using hits of pleasure to escape pain and it is controlling his life. I make one last impassioned pitch for rehab or a healing nature center. He declines, insisting he doesn't have a problem, which leaves me powerless. He is moving about 100 miles away, into the home of the most devoted grandparents on earth, Billy's parents. Once again, enabling will be disguised by love and devotion.

On January 1, 2013, Wilson packs a garbage bag full of clothes, his bull riding duffle bag, guitar, and bongo drums.

---

[7] For more insight, see Tara Heaton's TEDx talk, "Is Our Pleasure Killing Our Joy?"

Along with Tuff Amos and Sandy the non-detecting seizure dog, he backs his little red truck out of the driveway and heads for Memaw's house. He tells me he understands my decision and departs with his famous line, "Mom, I'm fine."

After Wilson moves in with his grandparents, I find myself better equipped to focus on Holly. She also copes with stress and grief by running, which again is probably a learned response. Her running has been into the wrong places or with the wrong people at times, but she primarily runs toward distraction with an over-booked calendar of work, social, athletic, and academic activities.

She is slightly more at ease now, knowing her brother is not going to call her to come get him in the middle of the night or show up at one of her high school parties drunk, behaving as if he has one night left to live. My lack of availability in her life has forced her to be independent and capable beyond her years, but that doesn't mean she has not been wounded by it.

I plan to take her last five months as a high school student to make up for even a sliver of the years of not giving her the mom I wanted her to have. We talk about her mental health, her regrets, and her dreams. We laugh remembering her first attempt at choosing a career for the future. She was a conflicted little five-year-old who declared, "When I grow up, I can't decide for sure, but I either want to be a Hollywood actress or work at the Golden Pantry." I bubble inside at the memory of such an innocent dreamer.

Now we are talking about college and a career in journalism. She wants to go far enough away where she is not defined as Caroline's sister or Wilson's sister but is free to be Holly. She has been accepted to the University of South Carolina. It's where she wants to go, but the out-of-state tuition is too costly.

I'm walking up the driveway, sorting through the mail. There is something from USC. I tear into it and read the news. Holly has been awarded a scholarship that more than covers the non-resident portion of tuition. I run into the house and up the stairs to give her the good news. As I bust into her bedroom, she is getting dressed and I see there is something on her ribcage. It's black. It's a— Oh no, it's not. Yes, it is. It's a tattoo.

"Holly! What have you done?" I bark. "I told you; you are too young for a tattoo! They can be addictive and one day you will totally change whatever it is you think is powerful enough to sear into your skin. But you will be stuck with it, branded with it forever! Holleeeee!"

She throws on her dad's old UGA sweatshirt and says, "Mom, chill. It's one tattoo. And I will never regret it."

I prop my hand on my hip, "And how can you be so sure? What does it say?"

She pulls the sweatshirt up and tilts to the side so I can see the cursive letters inked into her skin. I read it as she repeats the words aloud:

"I simply adore you."

Caroline is having what is called minimal breakthrough seizures. She may have one or two in a day, but will then go for up to three weeks without a single event. And the seizures are no longer tonic-clonic, the violent jerking type. They are milder, partial seizures[8] that may generalize into tonic seizures[9]. In comparison, this feels like a big win.

Due to her somewhat stable state and the fact that after eight years of epilepsy, Caroline has never had a seizure that didn't stop on its own, we make a change. I have conceded to letting her sleep alone. She moved into the bedroom closest to mine and sleeps in a queen bed that sits low to the ground. After so many years of sleeping with her mother, even this small taste toward independence gives her a sprinkle of renewed confidence.

It's Friday night, February 15, 2013. Holly is staying with a friend. I stop to kiss Caroline goodnight, make sure she is resting soundly in the center of the bed, and head to my bedroom. Ah. My room has become my little haven for peace. I love climbing into my own bed, all alone where I can find space for my thoughts to tumble as they please. There is a landline phone right by my head, but other than that, it is space and serenity.

I talk on the phone with Mike about the long days he is putting in at his new job. Caroline and I plan to drive to see him tomorrow. We will leave after breakfast and be in Greenville by lunchtime. We say goodnight, I switch off my lamp, and drift into a deep sleep.

---

[8] Partial seizures start in one half of the brain, and usually come with a warning that helps others to get the person to safety. This is unlike tonic seizures, which cause a sudden crash to the ground. See hopkinsmedicine.org for more information.

[9] This terminology was updated in 2017. Today these seizures would be classified as generalized motor or non-motor episodes. See: https://www.epilepsy.com/stories/2017-revised-classification-seizures.

The phone. The phone! The phone is ringing. I fumble to pick it up and squint at the alarm clock. It's 3:00 a.m. I think, *Wilson again*, and my heart starts to race. I answer with a groggy, grumpy hello.

"Is this Mrs. Heaton?" a strange voice asks me.

I confirm it is.

"You are the owner of an older model red Mazda truck?" the man asks.

"Um yes," I say sitting up. "It's my son's, actually."

"And do you know where your son is?" he asks.

I tell him I assume he is in Cartersville because that is where he lives now.

The man tells me he is with the Athens-Clarke County Police Department. He found Wilson's truck in a parking lot, but no one is in it. And then he says, "There has been an accident. We believe your son was driving and struck a young woman who was walking."

"Oh my God," comes out of my mouth. "Is she okay?"

My eyes squinch tightly as I tell myself to wake up from what must be a dream. I'm in a trance-like state that keeps me from processing words with clarity.

The man tells me the young woman is fighting for her life, but they don't know the extent of her injuries. He explains he is calling because they are looking for my son. He asks if I have heard from Wilson or know where he is.

It's so hard to think. I ask myself again if I have talked to Wilson and calmly verbalize the truth, "No. I haven't heard from him."

The officer tells me to try to reach my son and tell him they need to talk to him immediately. He says Wilson should come straight to the police station. He then gives me his number, which I try to remember in this dark state of shock, and we hang up.

I start calling Wilson's phone. Over and over again. I go downstairs to make coffee and keep trying. No answer. Finally, I call Billy. He agrees to head to my house and we keep trying.

The police officer calls again. He's not so patient this time. He insists I know where Wilson is. I tell him I have been trying to reach him. My thoughts are frozen in the present. There is no space to imagine what happened, where Wilson could be, or what we are facing. I'm a mechanical shell of myself, surviving each minute by avoiding the intense glare of reality.

The sun is coming up and Billy arrives. We sit at the kitchen table where we once used to sit as a family of five.

My phone rings from an unknown caller and I answer. It's Wilson.

My robotic mode takes over, forcing out perfunctory words, "Oh my God, Wilson! Where are you? What happened? The police called. They say they have your truck and that there has been an accident. You hit a young woman—"

I catch my breath.

Wilson responds, "What? I hit a person? Oh my God. I didn't see anything. I knew I hit something. It was loud. I thought maybe a deer. I don't know, Mom. I panicked. I parked my truck, and I have been sitting in the woods."

We find out that Wilson finally walked to a friend's apartment after several hours. *He's running. Always running.*

Billy goes to pick up Wilson and I stay home with a sleeping Caroline. At some point, I must have called Mike, because right after Billy leaves, he walks in. I don't get up. With an expressionless face, I stare at him. He walks toward me, pulls me out of my chair, and takes me into his arms. My arms remain pressed to my sides, extensions of the frozen, colorless mound of matter that is me.

When they return home, Billy tells Wilson to go get a shower and then we will take him to the police station. And in this moment, I say something I will forever regret. "Billy, no. I think we need a lawyer. We are all in shock. We don't know what we are doing."

He agrees that makes sense and calls a family member who works for a defense attorney. The lawyer, Jimmy, calls us immediately and tries to put our minds at ease. He calls the police for us, which I trust is a good idea. It is not. It makes it look like we are hiding, conniving. Wilson ran. And now it looks like we are trying to hide from the truth. Billy, Wilson, and I all agree we will be nothing but truthful. But I still think we should trust in our legal system, listen to a lawyer, and not just hand our son over with no representation.

Jimmy calls us back and says they don't want Wilson with a lawyer, that either he comes alone or they don't want him. Jimmy tells us to talk to no one. He says they have no proof Wilson was driving that truck and until they get it, they can't arrest him. However, he also says that we should prepare for them to show up anytime to take Wilson away.

"As soon as they have what they need, they will come to arrest your son."

I again tell Jimmy, no lying or covering up the truth. He says he understands, but we also can't be foolish. Wilson should not be talking to the police without a lawyer present. That makes sense to me.

I try to assess all that I have learned. Wilson told us he had been drinking, but not very much for his standards, because he was trying to impress a girl who was working at a bar. He was hungry, so when the bar closed, he went to get a few hotdogs and was going to call for a ride. He then thinks, *I'm fine,* and decides to drive. He said he was coming around the curve and never saw anyone.

I want to see the site and the truck. Mike drives me first to the weapon, the little red truck that I bought that has nearly killed a young woman. It has already been removed and impounded. So we head to the place where my son's truck struck a girl the age of Caroline, a girl who is in a coma, fighting for her life. We park and walk to where the accident took place at about 3:15 this morning. I try to stand on the little strip of grass that tilts toward the road, but it's too dangerous. I back away and inspect the yellow tape, the blood splatters, and the police markings where they retrieved her.

I am depleted, only able to will myself to perform movements that are normally automatic. I tell my foot to step into Mike's car. I tell my hand to reach over and close the door. As I watch my fingers secure the seatbelt, I remind myself to breathe. With my hands gripping the seat of the car, I continue to stare forward and say to Mike, "I want a pack of cigarettes. Please stop at a store."

"No! No, you don't want that."

With zero emotion, I simply state, "Either you stop, or when we get home, I get in my car, drive back to the store, and buy them myself." He stops.

We get home. I call Kathleen and tell her to come now. She arrives with wide eyes and sits without speaking. I smoke. I talk. She listens. I don't ask for a response; I just report the facts. She doesn't give me the clutch-and-tilt, she doesn't pity me, she just listens as she lets her tears trickle to a quivering chin. She doesn't tell me she is with me; I already know.

As days go by, my bleary eyes and shocked heart are glued to the news of the victim. She makes little progress. The torment I feel for her parents takes me back to January 2005. I can see myself and I know what they are doing. Laying their heads on the over-bleached, white banket that covers their motionless daughter, they are swimming in the beeping, clicking confines of shock and disbelief. They are begging, begging God to wake up their precious daughter. This image consumes me.

Wilson is staying with Billy. He pleads every day, wanting to turn himself in. The lawyer offers to bring him in to the police station, but they decline and say, "We have no warrant." They won't talk to him with a lawyer, and we agree that Wilson should not go alone. The detectives continue to search for the proof they need to arrest him.

Reporters and investigators swarm us every day. They walk into Holly's place of work and humiliate her while she is trying to fill pizza orders. While I'm worthless at work, letting Brad do my job, they even go to our house and try to interview Caroline.

Each day I remind Jimmy that we are not hiding from the truth. On week three of this torment, he has an idea and we agree. He offers that Billy and I give our statements based on what Wilson has told us. The detectives agree to two separate interviews, even with a lawyer present as long as he stays silent. Jimmy says after those interviews, the state will have what it needs to arrest our son.

We go down to the station and individually recount the morning of February 16, 2013, including Wilson telling us he knew he hit something or someone, and then parked his car and ran to the woods. In little more than an hour, the officers are at Billy's front door, with an arrest warrant for Wilson. He is booked and put in a jail cell. As impossible as it feels to accept, it's almost a relief. We knew this day would come. The waiting was torture, and surely unimaginable for the girl's family. For the weeks to follow, Wilson remains in a cell, awaiting the preliminary court hearing.

CHAPTER 39
THE POWER OF HEARTACHE

Same old porch, same old chair, same old ashtray. For the next two weeks, I sit, smoke, and try to try.

The birds are celebrating springtime as the sun starts to light the day. My shaky hand puts the cigarette to my lips as I wonder if I will ever kill this nausea and be able to eat more than three bites of a meal. This is a unique type of nausea, yet it's familiar. It's a distant memory, but yes, it's vivid and clear. I used to walk around with it as I fought Caroline's fate. It almost disabled me, rendering me useless to the world.

As it consumed me, I learned to use its energy to live in a perpetual combat mode, fighting off grief, softness, or any allowance of joy. But I learned to stop fighting off the pain, to let it in, repurpose it, and carry it back out into the world with love and wisdom.

Clarity warms through me. My flame meets the rising sun as I remember, I can't win this war. There is no fighting this attack on my heart. It floods my head with a weary, smoky cloud that sends tidal waves of nausea rolling inside me. I know this feeling because I have tried to battle it before. And in this moment, I realize, I know exactly what to do with it. I cannot waste its power.

I crush the unfinished cigarette, drop the box of Marlboro Lights into the ashtray and dump the entire symbol of helplessness into the garbage can. As I turn to head back into the house, I pick up speed and dash up the stairs. In record time, I'm in my car, headed north to Franklin County High School. They are waiting for their sophomore class to be dazzled and motivated by a speech that Brad is planning to give in my place.

Driving to the event along beautiful country roads, I remember one of the first times I ever stopped for a sales call at Franklin County High School. As I was leaving, I ran into a woman with a big, branded name badge. I knew it was my competitor's wife and smiled shyly as our eyes met. In her very southern drawl she said, "What are *you* doing here? This is *our* school."

As I pull into the parking lot today, I chuckle and think, *not anymore, Sugar.*

Four women greet me with the clutch-and-tilt at the front office. The news of Wilson is all over the state, so the staff, now treasured friends, are eager to hug me, comfort me, and pray with me. I am soft, open, and welcome their love. I express my gratitude and head to the auditorium where 400 sophomores have filed into seats, fidgeting, flirting, and jabbering while they wait. I head to the front as my steps spring in tandem with the booming pop music. Behind the stage I find Brad, sitting on a stool, microphone in hand, ready to greet the students. He looks at me, tilts his head just slightly and asks, "How ya doin', Tara Belle?"

A wide grin spreads across my face, I hold out my open hand and say, "Give me the fucking mic!"

For a few seconds, I close my eyes and ground into the reality that I have been entrusted with the next 30 life minutes of these students, each of whom is someone's precious child. The music fades, the curtains open, and the lights go up. Only because of the force with which I love, heartache burns like fire inside me. With my faithful fighting spirit, I transform that energy and step forward to give it away.

EPILOGUE

A BONFIRE

> "If it's painful, you become willing not just to
> endure it but also to let it awaken your heart
> and soften you. You learn to embrace it."
>
> — **Pema Chödrön**
> ***Start Where You Are: A Guide to Compassionate Living***

December 1, 2014

In Greenville, South Carolina, I sit up in the bed, inside the home that I now share with Mike. I hear him in the kitchen as I place my feet on the rug, and stare at its massive blue and green wildflowers. Usually I keep moving, but today I am fixated on my feet. I outline the big petals with my toes, ignoring the slightly chipped silver-gray polish. Smiling faintly, I think about how Caroline asks me about the bones protruding on my feet. She asks if they hurt. I tell her no. But she will ask again.

Today I see the feet that catapulted me off a diving board and never let me forget who has the ultimate power over my spirit. Today I see the feet that twirled my young frame into countless pirouettes, the feet that I crammed into cheap heels during my college years. I see the feet that walked me down the aisle to Billy, and the feet that steadied me as I lifted children, car seats, luggage, and baggage in and out of a Ford SUV for more than 20 years. These are the feet that walked me into Chipper's house to meet the love of my life. These are the feet that let me dance in the kitchen with my children; and these are the feet that helped me to run, run from pain, and run toward freedom. I stop swirling. I point my toes, relax them, and place them firmly on the ground.

Today these feet will lead me into the courtroom with my son. They will help me push past local reporters and face a severely injured young woman, her family, the judge, and Wilson's sentence. We have been anticipating this for 653 days.

And still I sit. I sit with the ache that is deep inside me. I don't fight it. I don't tell myself it's fine. It's not fine. It's sickening, that weighted nausea. With my hands in my lap, I invite the pain in and let it wash through me. And with a massive breath, I use it to propel me off the bed and get ready to face the reality of today.

As I slip behind the steering wheel to leave, Mike asks again, "You are sure? You don't want me there?"

I try to reply, but my quivering bottom lip just screws up my face, so I nod. I jump back out of the car, soak in my Germany's embrace one more time, and drive away.

When I arrive in Watkinsville, Wilson is waiting. Tuff

Amos at his feet, his guitar under his arm, his eyes clear, soft, full of fear. "Remember," I say into his eyes. "Remember our plan. You and only you can bring good from this. Few have done it. You will be one of the few. You will use this time, every minute of every day to learn and to grow."

In predictable Wilson fashion, he hugs me and tells me I'm the greatest mom in the world.

"Well, I do know this," I continue. "You are my son. Your spirit, your energy, your dedication to experiencing life with all your might, that is for sure me. And so, remember that. Remember the fighting spirit."

We both smile. And he says, "Mom, I could never forget the fighting spirit. You have been talking about it all my life. It's always with me."

As I watch Wilson say goodbye to Tuff, I wonder if a heart can in fact break. But I know mine won't. Today this heartache will burn solely as a source of strength and love for my son.

When we walk into the courtroom, I see the injured young woman and her family. These parents lost their only child, but this new daughter exists in her old familiar body. My hurt for them reaches a depth I didn't know existed. I want to hug her mom, tell her I feel her pain, her horror, so deeply. I want to tell her I know, I know your daughter is gone, yet she's here every moment, reminding you of who she used to be and all she dreamed of that will never be. I want to just sit with her and let her know. Oh, how I know.

The proceedings are brief because Wilson agreed to a 20-year sentence, 10 of which he is to serve in state prison.

Before the judge considers the sentence, Wilson is asked if he has anything to say. He stands up and turns to the devastated family. With a quiet voice that shakes with each word, he says, "I am truly sorry. I'm so very sorry."

The judge accepts the sentence and I watch Wilson stand. He is put into handcuffs and physically guided toward the back door. I say out loud, not caring who hears, "I love you, Wilson. You stay strong. We are with you."

He disappears. With a trance-like stare on my face, grief moves me methodically out of the room.

Warm tears flow down my cheeks as I drive back home in silence. I'm thinking of our first little rental house in Watkinsville. I smile through my tears, remembering the Christmas of 1998. Billy and I had worked hard to save for the big surprise. There was one small package under the tree addressed to all three kids, with the instructions to save it for last. Wilson opened it to find the little picture book I had made. He read each page aloud, and as the excitement built, so did their anticipation. When he read the last page, which said, "WE ARE GOING TO DISNEY WORLD!!!", Wilson, Caroline, and Holly erupted with joy, celebrating with the unbridled purity of children.

Those innocent babies are gone. Wilson is gone for now, stripped of his vices, left to face himself. Caroline's dreams are gone, and we have new dreams to reach. Holly is gone to college, hoping to find her voice, one that need not express trauma to be heard. This coming Saturday, Holly turns 20.

I will take the next few days to grieve. I will take time to dote on Caroline. And then on Saturday, I will drive to Columbia and give all of my love and all of my energy to celebrating the day Holly was born. We will laugh and dance. We will remember and we will cry. I will tell the story for the hundredth time, that has become our little ritual. And I will say, "I simply . . . " And she will reply, "*adore* you!"

As the night draws near, exhaustion swallows me. I slip into bed and place my cheek on Mike's chest, feeling his unfaltering strength and love. I try to speak, but he says, "Sleep, my Sunshine. Just sleep. I'm here."

I kiss him and my eyes fill with tears—tears born from hurt, from gratitude, and from love. My spirit will fight on. No fight is too tough for the bonfire that is love.

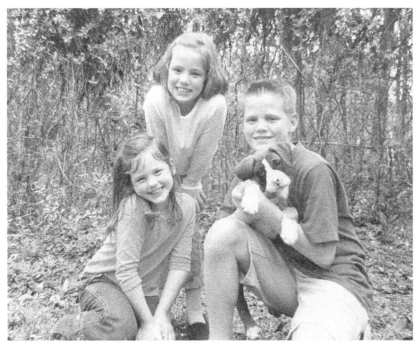

Clockwise: Wilson, Bruiser, Holly, Caroline. Year 2000.

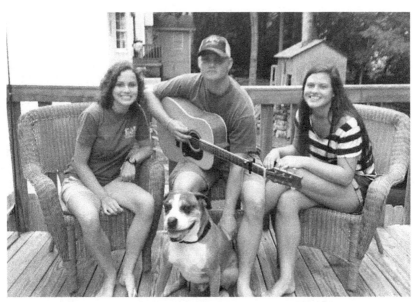

Clockwise: Wilson, Holly, Bruiser, Caroline. Year 2012.

ACKNOWLEDGEMENTS

WITH GRATITUDE FOR. . .

My father for making me a fighter and my mother for teaching me what to fight for.

Mike Noeth, for turning my life to full color, for seeing me as your sunshine in the rain, and for your faith in me as the author of this venture.

Holly Heaton, for inspiring eternal growth and for being the inextinguishable sparkler in my life. ISAY.

Caroline Heaton, for trusting me to keep hope alive and for teaching me to find treasures in moments that in any other life I would have missed.

Wilson Heaton for transforming my faith in human potential and for expanding my belief in the power of love.

Billy Heaton for being my trusted, forever family.

Kathleen Miller for laughter and for a soul-saving friendship.

Penny Treese for creating a book cover that personifies my spirit. Like your heart, your talent knows no bounds.

Team Caroline: Mary Brewer, Jeff Caldwell, Anthony Heaton, John Heaton, Pat Heaton, Kathleen Miller, Tim Miller, Jeff Rader, Lisa Thibault, Faye Warden.

The support of women who surround me with limit-less light and love: Dotsie Bausch, Mary Brewer, Celeste Cannon, Ginger Hiott, Holly Mims, Johanne Morin, Hella Noeth, Pat Nuzzaci, Kathryn Sabol, Laurie Shank, Rhonda Sillesky, Lisa Thibault, Penny Treese.

My original book coach and friend, Lisa Lilienthal, for being the first to help me believe we have a story that can elevate the human capacity for joy.

My publisher, Elizabeth Ann Atkins of Two Sisters Writing & Publishing. I talked to countless publishers, but when I met you, the search was over. You renewed my faith in hybrid publishing by putting art before business. For your passion, honesty, guidance, and vast wisdom, I am eternally grateful.

My editor, Trish Lockard of Strike The Write Tone. Thank you for pushing me, for teaching me the rules of a classic memoir, and then for putting up with my determi-nation to break those rules. Without you, this book would have been published as a mere collection of chronologi-cal memories written in story form. Thanks to your skill, passion, integrity, and tenacity, I trust we have a work of literature that can instill courage and ignite joy.

ABOUT THE AUTHOR

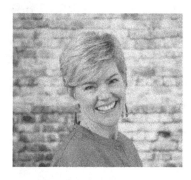

Tara Heaton combined her decades as a successful business owner and corporate sales trainer with her knowledge of neuroeconomics to create her company En Pointe Communication. Her study of the brain began as a relentless quest to cure her daughter's seizure disorder. Over time, it became an insatiable desire to learn more about memory, human behavior, habit, cognitive function, and neuroplasticity.

After years of research and with her sales and leadership experience, Tara developed her signature platform, Talk to the Brain™.

Talk to the Brain™ is designed to help teams and individual clients communicate for deeper connection and greater impact. It is the foundation for Tara's workshops, keynotes, and writing and coaching services that help clients tell unforgettable stories, improve results, and elevate joy through authentic communication. She teaches strategies and techniques based on what delights and influences the overstimulated minds in today's noisy world. Tara believes that the most crucial component of success at work and in life is our ability to create and elevate deep, trusting relationships.

To learn more about Tara's work, visit www.enpointe-global.com.

Enjoy her TEDx Talk, *Is Our Pleasure Killing Our Joy?* And check out her YouTube channel: @taraheaton3170.

To connect with Tara and learn more about the *Life Minutes* journey, please visit:

www.enpointeglobal.com/lifeminutes

https://www.instagram.com/taraheatonauthor

https://www.facebook.com/taracaldwell.heaton

To see photos from the *Life Minutes* journey, visit: www.enpointeglobal.com/lifeminutes

#lifeminutes

www.ingramcontent.com/pod-product-compliance
Lightning Source LLC
LaVergne TN
LVHW091507090525
810423LV00007B/3